Magic Mushrooms

The Beginner's Guide to Growing Magic Mushrooms

(Discover the Secret for Creating Your Own Garden in the Best Way Possible)

Robert Wasser

Published By **Bella Frost**

Robert Wasser

Magic Mushrooms: The Beginner's Guide to Growing Magic Mushrooms (Discover the Secret for Creating Your Own Garden in the Best Way Possible)

ISBN 978-1-998927-83-8

No part of this guidebook shall be reproduced in any form without permission in writing from the publisher except in the case of brief quotations embodied in critical articles or reviews.

Legal & Disclaimer

Table Of Contents

Chapter 1: History of Magic Mushrooms

Figure 2. Mayan mushroom stones one thousand B.C – three hundred B.C

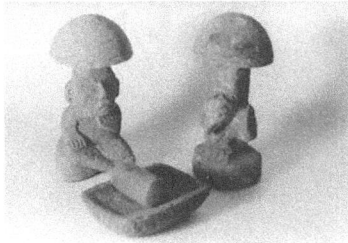

A TRIP BACK

The global's use of mushrooms extends decrease once more to Paleolithic times, or the Stone Age; a name given to the length amongst 2.Five million and 20,000 years in the past. Few humans recognize, or without a doubt don't want to do not forget, how influential the psilocybin mushroom has been in affecting the course of mankind's evolution. From easy tribal human beings in North Africa, to the 21st century non secular

1

excursion referred to as Christmas; we've had quite a adventure.

Figure 3. Cave painting Tassilli Algeria, 7,000

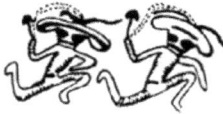

years in the past

Although the general information of magic mushrooms is purposely no longer pointed out, artifacts and artwork were observed to signify that mankind's love for psilocybin mushrooms dates as a ways lower returned as 7,000 years, in Tassilli, Algeria. However, it'd circulate once more even farther than that!

One idea via Terence McKenna is the Stoned Ape Theory. McKenna indicates that a number of the earliest identified human beings got here out of the jungle and into the grassland wherein they altered their food regimen. This new healthy eating plan consisted of mushrooms that grew from the dung of grass-grazing animals. The normal intake of psilocybin mushrooms are believed to have brought about big leaps in thoughts growth which in the long run superior mankind.

Whether these historic cultures were sincerely taking hallucinogenic mushrooms is up for debate. However, many indigenous tribes around the world exercise religious rituals with mushrooms these days.

One of the earliest written descriptions of the usage of psilocybin mushrooms comes from a Franciscan Monk named Motolinia (ca.1541). Motolinia modified into living with the indigenous tribes of South America. During this time period, the Spanish had been taking detail in their reign over the Americas.

"They had a wonderful approach of intoxication, that have worsened their cruelty, due to the fact inside the occasion that they took a few small mushrooms, they'll have a thousand visions in particular of snakes. They known as the fungi of their language Teonanacatl, what technique meat or flesh of the devil, they worship and in this way they have been led thru the bitter-tasting agent to their cruel god. "(Schultes & Hofmann, 1980)

Humans will preserve to consume magic mushrooms. Mushrooms are influencing records via innovation and could continue to inspire us even as we need it most. Yet nevertheless, all of those facts are not quite as thrilled because the magic that happened

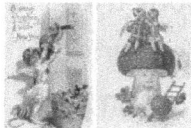

to tale of Christmas.

Figure 4. Merry Christmas!

THE MAGIC OF CHRISTMAS

You probably wouldn't be given as actual with me if I advised you that Santa (St. Nicholas), stockings, Christmas wooden, and reindeer had been all interconnected with the magic mushroom. Don't assume so? Just check the pics above. These are from the late 1900's. Pictured right here is the well-known Fly Agaric. This particular magic mushroom has a unique place in this Christmas story.

We begin in Russia with St. Nicholas, the Patron Saint of Russia. He is the second one maximum famous Saint nice to the apostles. Santa Claus, as maximum realize him, is a nickname given to St. Nicholas. It has been placed that in Siberia and the Arctic regions of Asia, the non secular shamans may go out into the wild to select out mushrooms.

Some shamans would likely put on religious garb that emerge as crimson, with white fur trim; especially much like the outfit worn by way of the use of Santa Claus. Others wore clothing along with the gadgets pictured under. They wore those shades as a tribute to the mushroom they have been looking; the Fly Agaric. When the shamans went on their lengthy trips, their yurt fashion houses might emerge as snowed in. This forced them to go through an opening in the roof (image a chimney). The modern-day day

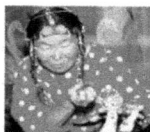

Santa Clause changed into born.

Figure five. Siberian Shaman

The shaman need to location the mushrooms in his bag near the fireside to dry, just like a Christmas stocking. Once dried, the shamans could provide them as gives, or offers, inside the path of the wintry weather solstice.

The maximum exciting proof of the psilocybin mushroom's have an effect on at the Christmas tradition come to be a non secular animal that modified into sacred to the shamans: the reindeer. In order to consume the fly agaric, the shamans may once in a while feed the raw mushroom to the reindeer. After ingesting the mushrooms, the reindeer would possibly jump wildly within the air as though they were flying, due to the powerful hallucinogenic.

Shamans might then acquire the urine from the deer with the resource of melting the saturated snow, and drink the liquid. The reindeer could reduce the toxin to consistent levels to allow hallucinogenic and non secular reviews for the shamans. Is the story beginning to come into awareness? It doesn't prevent there. You can't have Christmas without the gives, right?

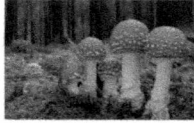

Figure 6. Fly Agaric

In his ebook, Mushroom and Mankind, James Arthur elements out that the Amanita Muscaria, moreover called fly agaric, "is usually discovered below birch and conifers within the northern Hemisphere. A conifer tree with some fly agaric underneath positive has a placing resemblance to a Christmas tree and offers."

Lastly, this all takes region within the northern hemisphere, in which it's cold and snowing. That sounds loads similar to the North Pole. So as you could see, it's tough to argue that there are documented information surrounding the genesis of Christmas. The tale that Santa and his reindeer must fly isn't always most effective a fairy story. Add within the stockings and the affords and we are not genuinely talking about a coincidence. Who may have idea the very aspect maximum oldsters were celebrating all our lives ought to have possibly been began via some small pink magic mushroom in Siberia!

Chapter 2: Mushroom Science

THE BASICS

To be a steward of a achievement mushroom cultivation, you should start with the basics. Knowing a number of the technology at the back of the mushroom will come up with a information base that you may in the end use to remedy troubles down the street. First, permit's begin with the life cycle of a mushroom.

Spores are mushroom seeds that first begin to germinate beneath first-rate situations. Individual X and Y Hypha are what sprout from the spores. As soon as one X Hypha connects with a Y Hypha, they create little one mycelium. You want both X and Y! If, as an instance, there have been to be five Y's, you wouldn't get mycelium.

After the mycelium consumes vitamins, the primordia paperwork. This need to arise within the right situations. This is the earliest recognizable degree of improvement of a fruit frame, aka mushroom. Finally a small coloured mushroom head will emerge and clearly mature to seed spores once more, as a

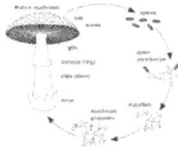

result completing the cycle.

Figure 7. Life Cycle of Mushroom

All mushrooms species have abortions, or aborts for quick. These are undeveloped fruit our our bodies very much like their vegetable cousins. The plant, or in this situation the mushroom, involves a selection that it's going to most effective produce a tough and rapid quantity fruit. The relaxation are aborts which can be decomposed via way of manner of nature. They are plenty smaller in length at the same time as in evaluation to a complete

11

grown mushroom. This makes them very smooth to recognize.

Lastly, mushrooms include over 90% water and the last 10% is crafted from fiber, proteins, vitamins and minerals. The developing may be categorized into three periods: Incubation, pinhead formation, and cropping. Even despite the fact that there are a few variations in species, the overall technique is pretty similar. We will go to the right conditions for the psilocybin mushroom subsequent.

THE CONDITIONS

Incubation duration: This is the period when you have inoculated your substrate (or grow medium) with spores and located them in a warmth, darkish place for you to germinate and change into healthy mycelium.

Temperature 28-30°C   (eighty two-86 °F)

Total darkness

Humidity ninety seven-one hundred %

Fresh air exchange: 0

Period: 2-four weeks

Pinhead formation: The duration even as you area the mycelium in oblique daytime and a decrease temperaturefor the first time. The mycelium will begin to shape the primordia. The mushrooms of their smallest usa are referred to as pinheads.

Temperature 22-24 °C   (71-seventy five °F)

Indirect sunlight hours

Humidity ninety-a hundred %

Fresh air exchange: 0

Period: five - 10 days

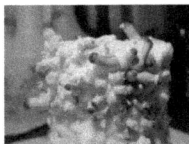

Figure eight. Photo of Pining

Cropping: After the number one pinheads have shown up, it is time for cropping. Cropping takes area even as the species grows into large fruit our bodies. This is also the time wherein you can see the aborts. A lot of glowing air and relatively low humidity are favored if you want to advantage achievement right right here. If no fresh air is exchanged, the mushrooms can be deformed. If deformations do upward thrust up, be sure to remove them to gain perfect effects.

Temperature 22-24 °C (71-seventy five °F)

Indirect sunlight hours

Humidity eighty - 90 %

Fresh air alternate: 3 instances an afternoon

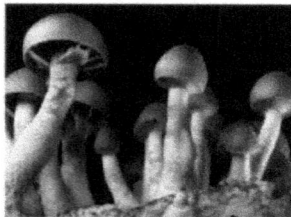

(minimum)

Period: three - 7 days

Figure nine. Spores release and fruit level, these mushrooms are geared up!

Chapter 3: MOLD

THE BASICS

Mold is your greatest enemy! You need to defend your life-style from being uncovered to mildew! Mold is a very unforgiving organism. Mold mycelium colonizes faster and their spores may be airborne in a don't forget of days; spreading just like the plague. Once you believe you studied mould, watch carefully. When you're sure it exists, put off it without delay thru carefully disposing of the contents of the jar. Place the contents into a plastic bag OUTSIDE within the trash.

For the most detail, mold is easy to pick out. It grows extremely fast! However, after a while, the mould turns coloration (A). If any of those sunglasses (green, blue, black or yellow) seem in the jar, DISCARD IMMEDIATELY!

NOTE: When the mycelium has been bruised, it turns a bluish coloration. This is not infection and has no effects for the first-class of the mycelium. But this picture underneath (B) illustrates a infected jar with blue inexperienced mould no longer bruised

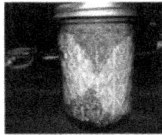

mycelium.

A.Figure 10. Yellow Mold

B. Figure eleven. Blue Mold

Lastly, while mycelium receives older it is able to start to form small yellow dots. This can also come to be a yellowish, slimy

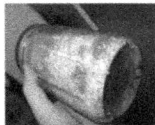

substance in a few times. This typically takes place with in reality colonized jars that have been inside the incubation length too prolonged. This is the harm-down of the substrate. That's not continually a awful factor. What IS awful is while the substrate is not liveable for the mycelium, see determine (A).

In this example, you'll see it develop spherical. These topics like to expand on shit. If they broaden round some aspect, it ought to be horrific. A properly rule to have a have a look at is:

When doubtful, honestly throw it out!

Chapter 4: Supplies and Prep

WHAT YOU NEED

In order to efficiently enlarge a crop of scrumptious shroomy caps, you need to observe the policies! With that stated, permit's get to it! You'll need to get the subsequent devices earlier than we get down and grimy.

• 10cc syringe (spores of a magic mushroom strain, companies on internet, chose biased at the exceptional opinions)

• One ½ pint jar (~240 ml)

• 140 ml vermiculite (Garden Center or Home Improvement Store)

• forty ml brown rice flour

• Extra vermiculite to fill the jar 1/4 inch from top

• forty ml water (boiled faucet or bottled spring water)

• Tinfoil (rectangular quantities will pass over jar mouth) or canning lid with 4 holes punched into the top. See figure 12 pg....

• 2 medium zip lock baggage (Grocery)

• Small metallic spoon

• Surgical gloves (Pharmacy)

• Mask (Pharmacy)

• Small 3 gallon plastic garage tub (Department Store)

• Plastic wrap (Grocery)

• Thermometer (It want to additionally diploma humidity)

• *Pressure cooker (non-compulsory and superb, but some different effective manner is using heat water tub so a three qt sauce pot with lid will do)

• Sanitation liquid (ethanol, vodka, or peroxide)

• Spray bottle (combined with a 50% sanitation liquid from above and 50% water)

• Measuring cups

• Paper towels

• Lighter

• Small ceramic plate

Most of those items want to be bought handiest as soon as and may be reused more than one times. Some devices might be already tucked away somewhere in your own home. If not, borrow them from a friend. Others may be bought at your community reduce fee maintain.

NOTE: Just make sure you operate 1 syringe in keeping with jar!

THE BASICS

Growing mushrooms isn't complex, but it's far touchy paintings. You will waste time and money if you do no longer comply with the ones easy, but crucial, commands. We will discover a very smooth and clean manner to expand magic mushrooms. There are many unique strategies to expand them, but for this unique ebook we may be focusing on one unique way.

Once you get the fundamentals down, you could improvement to greater difficult techniques. This will waste a top notch deal much much less time, cash, and emotion. So permit's have some achievement right right here, and then we're capable of flow directly to larger and higher.

THE RULES

Sanitation, sanitation, sanitation! The specific rule is endurance.

There are masses of masses of hundreds of micro organism, yeast and spores floating within the air that are not seen by using way of the bare eye. Just this form of little men can damage your entire task. You have to be cautious, so all utensils want to be sanitized first! Be overly essential approximately sanitizing. Next, have a chosen vicinity to your experiments to be completed.

THE PROCESS

Now allow's start. Right now you want three substances: brown rice flour (BRF), water, and vermiculite.

NOTE: Remember the 1:2:1 Ratio: 1 Part Brown Rice Flour, 2 factors vermiculite, and 1 trouble water.

There are many substrates to apply, but BRF is the maximum well-known. We might be the use of BRF for discussion skills. However, bird seed, manure, and distinct substrates have additionally been examined to artwork pretty well. In the prevent it's as masses as you, the cultivator.

STEP 1: You can purchase brown rice flour or grind 40ml of BRF to a flour consistency. You do that due to the fact the heat from the sterilization manner will kill the glaringly taking place yeast and mildew spores on the rice. (Leave apart – this will be delivered last.)

STEP 2: IN A BOWL, combine the 40ml of water and 80ml of vermiculite.

STEP 3: Once the vermiculite has absorbed the water, upload the BRF. Mix very well until in fact covered.

STEP four: Take a spoon and thoroughly scoop the mixture into the Mason jar. Once 1/2 entire, select out the glass up and faucet the lowest on a difficult floor. This will lightly p.C. And even out the combination.

NOTE: Don't faucet too tough or it'll % the substrate too tight. It wants to be fluffy and now not dense.

STEP five: Fill up the relaxation of the jar until there is an inch left from the lip. Then take a number of the final dry vermiculite and fill the very last place until it reaches ¼ inch from top.

STEP 6: Take a few foil and decrease out small squares to cover the hole of the jar. This will help to hold out mold, yeast and plenty of others. Place one piece of foil over the hollow of your freshly poured substrate and firmly clinch the edges tight. Then location the alternative piece of foil on actually tight sufficient so that it may be removed later. (For a reference see discern thirteen on the quit of bankruptcy five)

NOTE: You have to use a Mason jar lid with four holes punched in at 12 o'clock, three, 6, and nine and simplest use one piece of foil for the quilt. This is as a whole lot as you. (see decide 12 in Chapter five)

STEP 7: Put the glass jar right into a strain cooker set at 25psi for 15 minutes. Let it relax over night time time time INSIDE the stress cooker.

NOTE: Pressure cookers may be volatile, be careful!

If you don't have a pressure cooker, you can place the jar in a warm water bathtub and boil for 1 hour. For that:

Step eight: Fill the pot with water to about 1 inch from pinnacle of an empty clean jar or simply diploma so you understand how lots water to fill pot. Turn on range to medium excessive and cowl. It should roll to boil in 10min or so. Now place your mushroom cake jar in water bath for 1 hour and leave lid of the pot off. Watch this carefully. You don't need water splashing all over the area, but you do want the boiling water in order to kill any unwanted organisms present, 212 °F or one hundred °C. Finally, cool the jar overnight.

Chapter 5: Part 2 Inoculation

THE BASICS

Once the jar has cooled to room temperature, visit your art work location for the inoculation method. The aim right right here is to discover an area in which there are not any drafts and that can without issues be wiped smooth. Some human beings have a separate room for pastimes, while others use their kitchen. Don't neglect a rest room. It may be a splendid choice, especially if you have an overhead exhaust fan.

Once you've got your place selected, take hold of your masks and allow's get to artwork. Did you pay interest me? GRAB YOUR MASK! It will save you bacteria from being unfold whilst you breathe.

Please take each precaution that we go through right right here; you don't need to waste all of your tough paintings. Sanitation is vital! Wear your gloves or wash your arms well. You have to furthermore spray the room with sanitation spray.

BOTTOM LINE: YOU NEED A CLEAN AREA!

THE PROCESS

STEP 1:   With protection precautions taken, pull the syringe tip out of its cap.

STEP 2:   Take a lighter and burn the pinnacle simply until it's far red heat; then allow it cool. There may be contaminants on it so you have to try this step! And be careful no longer to soften the plastic.

STEP 3:   Peel off that first layer of foil (carefully with out ripping). Take the syringe tip and poke the needle through foil carefully as close to the brink of the jar, one at 12 o'clock, one at 3, one at 6, and one at nine (as you're looking on the pinnacle). See image underneath for an concept.

STEP four: Follow the needle down on the aspect of the glass, almost as if you're scraping it. You want the bottom end of the needle (plastic detail) to be touching the foil.

NOTE: Be cautious not to tear the foil or you could need to start for the duration of. The smaller the holes, the higher off you'll be. You have to use a canning lid to avoid this with 4 holes. You though would possibly need to cover with a sheet of foil to maintain contaminants out after inoculation.

STEP 5:   Squeeze out simplest ¼ of the spore solution in each of the 4 holes. If accomplished correctly, you may see the solution unfold over the inner of the glass and run down the bottom. The maximum import element to do proper here is to hit the substrate (or cake) in identical elements with the spore answer. If you don't see this, you may threat the cake or substrate not sincerely colonizing.

NOTE: If you attempt to expand mushrooms with a partially colonized cake, you can get achievement. However, your cake will most likely best in part colonize, and also you'll chance mould or micro organism. Mold can short take over your cake. Remember, mold grows faster than mycelium!

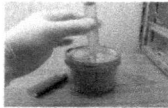

Figure 12. Inoculation

STEP 6: Take the piece of foil that you took off and vicinity it lower again over the outlet of the field and clinch the foil tight. Place it somewhere darkish and warmth (spherical seventy seven-82 °F or 25-27 °C).

NOTE: Above a refrigerator in cabinet is a excellent region, but anywhere will do that doesn't get moderate or high-quality temperature fluctuations.

THE RESULTS

It all is based upon in your spores at this factor. If you likely did the entirety effectively, you want to appearance a few mycelium growth as speedy as 2 days. However, it could take in to every week or so. Sometimes you may do everything right and it doesn't training session.

DON'T GET DISCOURAGED!

Earlier, we said that every species is one-of-a-kind. Some may also additionally colonize in 2 days and hold for multiple weeks, while others might likely soak up to a month. Some don't even expand the least bit. In this example it is most possibly client mistakes; or you can have supplied some horrible spores. Don't beat your self up if you aren't a hit the primary time. Mushrooms in trendy are very touchy. The best element to do is prepare them in batches and be privy to detail.

NOTE: Keeping a mag can be very useful.

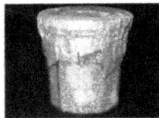

Figure thirteen. This is a fantastic signal after some days.

I apprehend how excited you'll be to see how your mushrooms are doing, however the awesome element to do is clearly to permit nature take its course. You don't want to test on them each day. Just take a look at every few days for mycelium growth. Once you notice some, you're golden! After that, there can be no want to test greater than as soon as every week. You don't want to threat mildew or micro organism outbreaks with the aid of dealing with them an excessive amount of.

Now, at the same time as the cake is in fact colonized, you have to be searching at a stable white cake of mycelium (See photograph beneath). If you notice some thing aside from white proper here (or a few difficulty that resembles mould), THROW IT OUT! I can't strain this sufficient! The ultimate detail you need to do is eat some poison loss of existence mould or breathe in the spores.

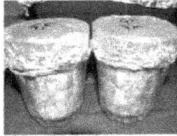

When unsure, clearly throw it out.

Figure 14. Fully inoculated

Chapter 6: Part 3 Fruiting and Harvest

THE BASICS

So, updated, you've accompanied the sanitation rules and protocol for inoculation. Now you're left with a nice white cake that is virtually colonized with psilocybin mycelium. CONGRATS! But you're not executed. Now you want a fruiting chamber. Let's live clean via using a few problem consisting of a plastic field. The critical topics to pay interest on proper right right here are: sanitation, mild, humidity, and pruning.

THE PROCESS

STEP 1: Take your 3 gallon box, plastic wrap, gloves, and mask from your deliver list. Go to your paintings place and sanitize EVERYTHING.

STEP 2: Take 50ml of dry vermiculite and pour into a pile inside the center of plate. (Wash fingers or placed on gloves). Then take your cake and punctiliously faucet it out onto the dish. This can also additionally moreover make an effort. Be cautious no longer to interrupt the cake.

STEP three: Place the cake with dish into your 10 gallon area. Place thermometer/humidity gauge in the corner. Take 2 tablespoons of water and positioned it on the lowest of your problem. This will increase humidity and prevent the cake from drying out. Now, cowl the sector setting up with a plastic wrap. A Double layer is probably proper. Make high nice to use a few quantities of tape to stable the plastic wrap so it doesn't glide off your field. It is important that the plastic stays consistent and acts as a barrier to keep dust, insects, or mould from inhabiting the field.

NOTE: three-5 times an afternoon you can bring the plastic wrap as lots as allow glowing air into the field. It doesn't need to be every few hours. It may be random.

Fresh Air in this diploma is important for correct mushroom boom.

THE CONDITIONS

LIGHT

It's truely an vintage better halves story that mushrooms don't want light; they absolutely do within the starting. Sometimes a small moderate is used, but not something near what a house plant desires. Dim room mild will art work certainly super. There's no need to have a special mild. The plastic wrap permits moderate to get to the substrate. That's all you want. The moderate tells the mycelium that it's prepared to fruit due to the fact they've reached the prevent of the substrate. Now they are able to reproduce, or in this case, release spores.

HUMIDITY

The humidity wants to be at ninety%. If it gets to 100%, you can start to see issues.

Conversely, going underneath 75% will force the mushrooms to begin drying out earlier than they may be absolutely grown. The sweet spot is eighty five-ninety% humidity.

WHAT TO LOOK FOR

With the proper moderate and humidity, the regular length is -4 days till you begin to see little clusters of white pin heads forming. The day after this takes location you need to look brown heads (See picture in financial disaster three). Mushrooms will double each day. The temperature wants to be among 78 to eighty 4°F, 25-29 °C. Different species can tolerate levels in temperature, however normally, that is the median variety. The breakdown of a nutrient rich cake creates a small amount of heat. So to avoid big fluctuations, you could wrap the lowest of the field with a bath towel to help with warmth retention.

Sometimes whilst mushrooms sprout out they will forestall growing. Others will keep to double in duration. You need to prune the small mushrooms. These mini mushrooms are the aborts that we cited in bankruptcy 2. The real mushrooms must be distinguishable through manner in their boom in assessment to the aborts. You can also see aborts come first, however ultimately you harvest the massive ones.

NOTE: Do not devour aborts! Pick them out and throw them away. If you don't, they'll curl up and turn blue or gray. This is but each other way for mold and bacteria to thrive. They're moreover eating precious nutrients, so simply cast off them right away! In the give up the harvest, or flush quantity, might be four-eight massive mushrooms developing at a time. However, this really depends at the species. There can be greater (which is generally higher).

HARVEST

The time to harvest the mushroom is simply earlier than the veil (the skinny membrane underneath the cap) exposes its gills. Once the gills are uncovered, they quickly drop their spores. However, it's far superb that you harvest a touch faster; ideally while the cap remains in a ball-like form. You should pick out out them later, however they may make a mess on the identical time because the spores drop.

The right way to pick out out a shroom:

• Have smooth arms or put on gloves

• Wear your mask

• Gently pinch close to the bottom and slowly twist till the shroom offers manner.

NOTE: Every time you have were given contact at the facet of your cake, you danger contaminating it!

Your mushrooms will look better at the same time as you pick out them in advance. If you're considering letting them expand to increase psilocybin and psilocin tiers; don't problem. The ranges max out half of manner via its fruit cycle. Looking at the image underneath, some of those were left a day too lengthy. However, in case you are collecting spore prints, it's an excellent time.

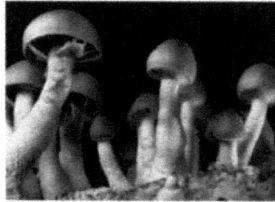

The mushrooms on the lower right of the image are near best. That's what you want. Technically, possibly even a 12-24 hours earlier. The mushrooms at the left are too far lengthy past. These is probably perfect for accumulating spores prints despite the fact that. Nevertheless, as long as you select them in advance than the caps curl up and drop spores, they're all nicely to reap.

Figure nine.

SECOND FLUSH

After the mushrooms have long gone through one entire growing degree, don't throw away the cake or substrate. Let it rest for two days in a darkish location. Once the cake has rested, put on gloves and a mask, and sanitize your artwork place. Next, do away with the cake from the terrarium after which wash and sanitize it. Fill it with three inches of water. Place your cake laying on its component within the water bath. Place the washed ceramic plate on top of your cake carefully.

NOTE: For water bath, you should purchase bottled water or put together by means of way of boiling faucet water to rid any possible contaminants and remove the chemicals. Then, permit it cool to room temp. You also can positioned 1-2 tablespoons of peroxide in the water. This will assist combat any contaminants as nicely.

The cake needs to soak in a water bath at room temperate in a single day. This is wanted because of the reality the cakes are dense, so that they require a complete 24 hours of soaking. This way will permit them to soak up more water and be prepared for some other fruiting.

HOW TO TRIPLE YOUR YIELD!!!

The cake is rich in nutrients. After a few flushes, you could experience much like the cake is completed. However, you could get many greater flushes out of the substrate in case you without a doubt top off the moisture and allow it relaxation a couple days in amongst. It's very viable for your cake to offer mushrooms for up to eight flushes or more if you comply with this technique! They gained't be as massive as the first few, however all of it counts.

Chapter 7: Drying and Storage

There are some outstanding methods to dry your mushrooms, but we'll start off with the correct (and I trust the pleasant). The reason is to dry them as definitely as feasible. Drying too quickly must disturb the efficiency. Drying too gradual can also need to motive mildew. There are many methods to dry your bounty, but keep in mind the following manner first.

THE BASICS

The maximum easy and powerful way to dry your mushrooms is by using manner of the use of placing them on a bit of paper and leaving them someplace out of the way. What you're seeking out is the mushroom to be crispy. It wishes to lose its moisture for garage features. This process can also take a few days. You will see your mushrooms lessen again in duration.

NOTE: Remember that mushrooms are ninety% water. This is a totally natural way to dry so all the performance is preserved. Excessive heat for quick right away gratification would possibly harm your mushrooms.

The key's to keep away from moisture. If there is any moisture above three%, it will increase mould. So don't be too short to maintain them in that air tight subject. After a few days, check their development. To do this, take a stem and break it in 1/2 of. If it snaps like a sprig, you're in pinnacle form. Allow a pair greater days for the larger ones.

Now you're stable to preserve them in a pitcher jar with a rubber seal for long run. Or, you could dive right in and eat them proper away. For longer storage even though, keep a regular temperate among sixty 5 -seventy 3 °F, 18-23 °C.

OTHER METHODS

Another technique of drying and storage is accomplished by means of way of manner of the use of a warm temperature lamp (or oven) at low warmness 140 °F, 60 °C. A more steady manner might be to get a meals dehydrator. It's feasible to preserve your mushrooms longer through the usage of a vacuum seal bag and setting them in the freezer. This method has been set up powerful in keeping the performance.

Chapter 8: Collecting Spores

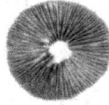

Figure 15. Spore Print

THE BASICS

Collecting your personal spores will save you a ton of coins! Each syringe can fee everywhere from 10-30 US Dollars. By acquiring and utilizing this data you don't should hold looking for spores (which will be unstable depending on your america's legal guidelines). Not quality does buying spores come to be expensive, you don't even realise if they're glowing. By supplying yourself you keep cash, boom extremely good, and limit your hazard.

Collecting spores is a terrific knowledge that you have to look at. To begin gathering your private spore prints, you have to depend on your experience of timing. Timing in truth is the whole thing on this method. To get an remarkable spore print, the mushroom need to be picked certainly because the veil has damaged and the cap has not but flattened out. Let's smash down the technique.

THE PROCESS

STEP 1: With easy arms (or gloves) take a easy picked mushroom and reduce the steam as near the cap as viable. If you leave an excessive amount of of the stem it'll get within the way and you gained't capture the most amount of spores.

STEP 2: Take a easy piece of tin foil and decrease a 3x3 rectangular.

STEP 3: Take the cap and vicinity it at the foil, gill side down.

STEP 4: Take a shot glass (CLEANED & SANITIZED) and region it over the cap. Place it someplace wherein it acquired't be disturbed.

NOTE: Wait days to get the first rate effects. After 2 days, there can be no significance in the quantity of spores that drop. The first 24-36 hours are the maximum ample. It must look exactly just like the photo above.

STEP 5: After days, cautiously improve the shot glass. Take the foil and carefully fold it into a rectangular, folding the rims so it's sealed.

STEP 6: Place the foil in a NEW zip lock bag and put it someplace fairly cool for storage.

NOTE: It will be prudent to hold some mushrooms for printing from each flush. Over the life of the cake you may have 10-20 prints for future use. And because you probable did it yourself, you recognize they will be the right stress and clean.

HOW TO MAKE A SYRINGE

THE PROCESS

STEP 1: Take an vintage or new syringe and sanitize the pinnacle with alcohol or thru flame.

STEP 2: Boil half of of cup water; preferably natural distilled water.

STEP three: Insert alcohol or peroxide into syringe filling 1/2 of way to kill another contaminants, and many others. For 5-10 mins. Then remove the liquid from syringe.

STEP 4: Take the boiling water and fill the syringe half of whole. Shake the syringe, then allow it sit down for 10 mins.

Repeat this technique 5 instances or so; essentially till the water has no trace of alcohol or considered one of a kind sanitizing liquids. You can check this through taste, but DO NOT SWALLOW.

STEP 5: Sanitize the stop one more time and fill the syringe with water unit it's entire. Place the cap over the pinnacle give up and allow it rest till it has cooled to room temperature.

STEP 6: Go to your artwork station and sanitize the place. Be nice to place on a mask and gloves.

STEP 7: Take the foil print out of the bag and thoroughly spread.

STEP eight: Take the foil and create a bowl-like shape but DO NOT DISTURBE THE SPORES! Then squeeze the water from the syringe over the spore print.

NOTE: You will see the spores begin to launch themselves. You can also need to apply the give up of the syringe to loosen the spores from the foil.

STEP nine: Once maximum of the spores have dissolved into the water, carefully suck up the spores into the syringe.

NOTE: You may also scrape them right into a clean shot glass the usage of a small clean knife, and following the same method with the water; both manner works nicely.

STEP 10: Flame the top, then permit it cool. Now positioned on the cap and maintain the syringe in a NEW smooth zip lock bag within the fridge. Don't neglect about to region a label on it!

NOTE: One way that is beneficial is to label the zip-lock with "Date" and "Strain".

Chapter 9: The Consumption of Mushrooms

When you're ingesting mushrooms for the primary time, it's endorsed which you start off with a low dose. It actually is predicated upon at the pressure of mushroom. Some are stronger than others, however it's far been typically widespread that 2 grams is ideal for a number one timer. Try 1.Five grams in case you're now not positive. You have to pass as heaps as 4 grams in case you are an professional shroomer.

NOTE: CAUTION IS WARRANTED!

Consuming mushrooms is a form of managed food poisoning. There is a hazard that you may get ill and probably vomit. If illness persists, devour a few activated charcoal. You can collect charcoal at the neighborhood pharmacy. If there may be continuous vomiting after half of-hour of charcoal, are in search of medical hobby right away!

Mushrooms are normally eaten right now after being dried, but in addition they may be ate up in a tea or thru manner of cooking them. Cooking will lower their efficiency due to the excessive temperatures. Eating glowing mushrooms is an preference, despite the fact that that is a excellent deal extra powerful and is NOT RECOMMENDED TO ANYONE!

Here are some ideas to get you started if you don't need to consume them without delay:

MUSHROOM TREATS RECIPES

Peanut Butter Bon Bon

Serves 1

1 Tbs Peanut Butter

2 g Dried Mushrooms

25 oz. Semi-Sweet Chocolate

25 oz. Dark Chocolate

Directions

1. Take mushrooms and ruin or reduce into small crumb like portions.

2. Then, combination the mushrooms chunks with warmed peanut butter till very well mixed. Take mixture and positioned it in freezer to sit back. (Don't freeze)

three. Melt chocolate in a double boiler (one pot full of boiling water with a bowl floating on pinnacle to save you burning)

4. Take peanut butter combination out of freezer and roll proper right right into a ball. Use a touch flour to help with stickiness.

5. Take peanut butter balls and dip them or roll them within the chocolate aggregate until lined. (Try a 2nd or 1/three coat).

6. Place on sheet pan covered with wax paper. Then hooked up fridge to relax.

7. Eat after chocolate has hardened. Store the rest, if any, in air tight subject

Mushroom Tea (Merlin's Elixir)

Serves 1

2 g of Dried Mushroom

10 ounces.. Water

3-four leaves of clean Mint

2-three paper-skinny slices of Ginger

2 Lemon twists (2 inches lengthy and .25 large)

1 tsp honey

Directions

1. Grind mushrooms to a powder (espresso grinder works properly)

2. Bring 10 ounces... Of water to a boil

three. Remove from warmth and allow sit down for five mins

four. Stir in mushroom powder in levels

5. Add mint, lemon twist, honey, and ginger

6. Let steep for five mins

7. Take out the massive chucks and watch for it cool

Enjoy!

Shroomy Pizza Bread

Serves 1

6 Inch extended piece of Italian Bread

1.25 fl oz.. Preferred Tomato Sauce

1/three cup Mozzarella Cheese (or desired cheese)

(Few pinches Parmesan Cheese non-obligatory)

2 g Magic Mushrooms

Directions

1. Cut the italian bread in 1/2 of of so that you have a bit 6" prolonged. Then lessen that piece in 1/2 of of lengthy way so all you

have got got left are halves. We are the use of simplest one issue.

2. Remove some of the get right of entry to bread inside the center to make a ship form. Toss get proper of entry to bread to the factor.

three. Take bread boat and lightly brush the hole space side brush with some olive oil.

4. Place under broiler under at 3 hundred °F or 148.89 °C until slightly golden on pinnacle. Remove and allow cool.

5. Take sauce and region right into a bowl. Crush mushrooms or depart whole with sauce and place it into the bread boat hole area.

6. Sprinkle cheese and oregano on top and region lower returned into oven below broiler till cheese is melted.

Take out, allow cool and revel in!

NOTE: It is extraordinary to eat magic mushrooms with a few pals and feature a plan. Once you've eaten the ones magic mushrooms, you've got made a strength of mind for the subsequent 4 hours. You could make a list of troubles you want to resolve, format a venture which you need to create, or clearly tap into that experience of spirituality. Whatever has you inquisitive about consuming magic mushrooms, just make certain you are inside the right mind-set. This manner warding off them if you're having a awful day!

Chapter 10: FAQ's

Can I use easy white rice or a few one-of-a-kind form of rice?

Brown rice has extra nutrients than your latest white rice. Mushrooms want those vitamins to expand, as a end end result making brown rice a superior substrate over white rice. Using brown rice in vicinity of white need to increase your yield.

Did I make a terrible choice of jar?

A large-mouth half of-pint (~234ml) is recommended for vermiculite and brown rice flour desserts. Larger jars will take longer, and may be less complicated to infect if too massive.

Is my substrate too wet?

If you saturate the aggregate an excessive amount of, you may both add a piece extra BRF or Vermiculite. You might also moreover microwave for a minute or exposed to evaporate the get proper of access to water. A appropriate tip to avoid this trouble is to wet the vermiculite first, till saturated, and then add the BRF.

My aggregate isn't ethereal and it looks as if dust

Use huge bite vermiculite, and do no longer shake or compress the substrate thru squashing it down. You will observe in the course of the technique that a small amount of air change is crucial to healthful mycelium boom. The extra you % the substrate, the lots less air there's available to it. You may additionally have used too much water as properly.

Is it viable to have an incomplete sterilization?

Always offer it greater time to ensure. If you're compelled to sterilize at a lower temperature placing, constantly upload extra time. Remember, if using a strain cooker, observe the suggestions! A golden rule is to permit the cooker come to pressure or at the identical time because the water is boiling, then begin timing.

Can you inoculate too fast?

Let the jars get to room temperature after boiling or stress cooking. Mycelium will die if heated to or above 106°F (41.1°C). Your fingers aren't high-quality temperature gauges, so do no longer inject spores until you're honestly sure they have got cooled. A appropriate rule is to permit it cool in a single day.

No pins even 10 days after starting the fruiting diploma?

Check your mild, temp, and air exchange. Inspect for infection and pests. Try to govern every aspect and you'll be positive. Go decrease back to preceding chapters of this e-book for reference at the manner to beautify your information.

How lengthy to develop?

Please be affected man or woman and do not panic after quality 2 days; irrespective of how rapid you bear in mind the colonization should be. After a time period and now not the use of a germination, check all of the opportunities that could keep away from the growth (i.E. Temperature, substrate, spore interest, and age of the spores). This is your pleasant bet on reading the details of your private setup.

Because there are such lots of tremendous relevant factors, it's very hard to decide inside the 1st or 2d weeks why you haven't visible germination. Give it as a minimum every week earlier than you worry, and at least 3 weeks earlier than you panic. All you want are 2 spores to germinate to take over the complete jar.

What is gasoline exchange?

When mushrooms digest a substrate, they produce carbon dioxide and consume oxygen. This is a fairly vital component determining the success of mycelium boom. There have to be at the least a small amount of air alternate.

What is the white fluffy stuff?

When there's too much moisture in the air the mycelium is able to develop outward. When the humidity is reduced, this want to move away. However, continually maintain the humidity close to the candy spot at ninety%. Also, watch closely for the possibility of mildew.

I virtually have little flies in my fruiting chamber. What do I do?

These are not flies. They are fungus gnats. They are the worst pest on the identical time as growing mushrooms! The possibilities of you saving your cake after see them are slim. The fungus gnats feed on mycelium or mould of every type. The woman can lay over 1,000 eggs of their existence time. You ought to throw out your cake(s) to ensure you get the adults.

Leave a bowl of oil out with some drops of apple cider vinegar. Place the bowl close to a desk mild in a single day, with the mild on. In a few days they will start death inside the bowl. You CAN NOT begin over again until for effective they've got all been disposed of. Just two of those guys can alternate into hundreds in a take into account of a pair weeks!

The spore's colonization went pretty rapid for few days, and then it suddenly stopped developing

Check the air trade. There possibly isn't enough glowing air attending to the colony. Also, take a look at your temperature and light. Remember, at this segment of way, there should be no slight. Most importantly, BE PATIENT!

I sold a 10cc syringe. Can I use it for more than one jar?

No. To acquire the notable opportunity for fulfillment, use one syringe for one jar.

Otherwise, you risk the cake now not colonizing all the manner. Then, in desire to saving on a syringe, you've lost the entirety else. Review financial disaster nine on a way to make a spore syringe.

Chapter 11: Where to enlarge your mushroom

Outdoor cultivation

Growing outside mushrooms are amazing in lots of methods because of the reality the forest (or any dreary location with appropriate humidity and air float) gives the proper fruiting conditions without the need of the farmer for any weather manage. In reality, the wooded area is wherein the mushrooms we increase come from, so why not truely increase them to be had? This is the concept which brought about the development of Cornell's initial mushroom research and extension assignment led through Professor Kenneth Mudge (now Emeritus), who have become especially interested by agroforestry, or the aggregate of bushes, forests, and crop manufacturing.

Ken has been analyzing many species for nearly 15 years, especially targeting log-grown shiitake mushrooms as they fast proved to have the most charge range excellent viability. We additionally understand that mane, oyster, wine cap Stropharia can be effectively grown outside, and a few remarkable minor species. The important limit with outdoor or wooded area cultivation is that only the log-grown shiitake can grow normally sufficient out of the species said above to deliver weekly mushrooms, a vital a part of the supply chain to a farm organisation organization. This is because of the precise property that shiitake logs can be soaked or "forced" into fruit thru immersing the logs in water for 12-24 hours, which inspires them to go through fruit. This device can be used to broaden instead constantly mushrooms from throughout the number one week of June via the middle to overdue part of October, at least in Central New York's weather. Although inexperienced, the other species produce fruit on their very personal, and so aren't proper selections if the intention is to yield constant market yields.

Indoor Growing

Once we step out of the woods and into an enclosed location, the list of species that we're capable of reliably develop begins offevolved to enlarge drastically. In addition, we must moreover start to expose and hold the first-rate environment for the incredible manufacturing levels, from incubation to fruiting. And possibly the maximum hard problem, we need to take extra measures to lessen and cast off contamination assets in our substrates, if you want to arrest and save you fruiting of our preferred mushrooms. With out of doors production, this hassle is form of non-existent, a massive advantage aspect. Indoor farming structures are on occasion known as "managed agricultural surroundings," which incorporates awesome structures together with hydroponics, aquaponics, and greenhouse production. Unlike CEA structures used for vegetables and herbs, mushrooms can be produced in places with confined infrastructure and assets for manufacturing start-up and sustainability. However, worries and controls need to be made concerning the prevailing temperature, humidity, slight, and airflow.

Chapter 12: Sterile way of existence approach

Mushroom food (well known as its substratum) is much like human meals: a nutritious combination that contains a stability of carbohydrates, proteins, minerals, and nutrients. Like our meals too, I discover a number of microorganisms quite fine, as a loaf of bread neglected in the kitchen counter will speedy show for a number of days. Unlike human beings, but, fungi are also micro-organisms and need to compete with some different community micro-organisms for food. Bacteria and molds have a competitive side because they might reproduce lots, even heaps and heaps of times faster than the not unusual species of mushrooms can. Any substrate that even includes a single mould spore or bacterium will possibly come to be a moldy or mild mess. Furthermore, within the commonplace room, the commonplace cubic centimeter of air incorporates greater than 100,000 particles. No count how scrupulously smooth you accept as true with you studied it's miles, an invisible, silent rain of mold spores, dust particles, and pollen grains settles constantly on each horizontal ground in your property. The only manner to prevent those critics from hijacking the mushroom cultures is to make certain that they in no manner get without delay to them first. There are popular techniques to do this: through jogging in a clearly clean (i.E., sterile) environment, they thoroughly kill some component molds or bacteria are there, to start with, and exclude some other. We extract pollution from our products through sterilizing them in a stress cooker, in which nearly no dwelling issue also can face up to the high temperatures (1210 C/ 255' F) and pressures (15 psi) inner them. We then create a sterile running environment through filtering the air in our workspace and/or the usage of chemical disinfectants to sterilize it.

Those strategies represent the method of sterile or aseptic farming, it actually is through manner of a long way the most critical component you need to recognise to attain cultivating the mushrooms. Let me reiterate this for emphasis: The maximum critical trouble you can have a look at from this e-book is the sterile life-style approach. If you do now not decide out this one, no longer one of the strategies of cultivation will artwork, irrespective of how carefully you comply with the instructions. If you're simply, really fortunate, you may possibly harvest one or two mushrooms, but in maximum cases you will have a glowing array of blue, inexperienced, and black molds and a slimy, pungent bacteria collection. Many could probably-be mushroom growers have failed proper proper proper right here, and people who succeeded (consisting of your humble authors) have found the difficult way of the use of sterile way of life strategies and why. It is our desire that the techniques supplied on this financial disaster will display you the clean manner, saving you time and heartbreak.

Cleaning your paintings region

The instruction of a clean workspace is the number one undertaking. Ideally, you could best dedicate a room or vicinity on your mushroom obligations, like a spare mattress room or an unused stroll-in closet. If there's no such space, then a exceptional deal of the laboratory paintings may be finished in a mean kitchen, but this calls so that you can installation and maintain a pristine stage of cleanliness. The kitchen competes with the relaxation room because of the truth the house's messiest and biologically energetic room, and the counts of molds there have a propensity to be very excessive. Working in a kitchen, however, affords reachable get right of access to to a water supply and furnace top. If you are planning to commit a separate place to mushrooming, make certain it is close to the kitchen. There's no thing in sterilizing your substances absolutely to hold them into your laboratory via a dirty residence. A accurate-sized table must be in the workspace, preferably one with a non-stop, with out problem wiped clean higher floor. Formica or enamel is proper because of the truth earlier than every use you could want to wipe the workbench with alcohol. If you have a wood table, maintain in thoughts setting on pinnacle of it a piece of skinny plywood with a plastic laminate floor, or a bit of heavy, thick vinyl at the same time as going for walks. Similarly, it have to be easy to smooth the workspace floor (linoleum or tile), and smooth to check out for cleanliness. Carpets are spores and dirt repositories, tens of loads of hundreds of which may be kicked into the air each step of the way and need to be averted if feasible. The partitions need to be smooth (a sparkling coat of paint couldn't harm), and any other room areas and surfaces need to be wiped clean thoroughly. Use a solution for disinfecting if practical (orange-oil based totally merchandise are nicely as they may be slight however effective biocides and environmentally nice). Obviously, if you paintings on your kitchen, you can't disinfect each surface whenever you plan to use it, however you need to however deliver it a ordinary deep cleansing and disinfect as an lousy lot of it as you can before every use. Space want to be void of drafts to decrease air pass spherical your cultures. Windows ought to be tightly closed, heating or air-conditioning ducts want to be blanketed, and doorways ought to be closed lengthy before you start work. Whenever possible get rid of special assets of infection from the room. Potted flowers, fish tanks, meals plates for pets, muddle bins: get all of them out of there. It is useful to run an air-filtration device in the area too.

Good ones in recent times charge lots a great deal much less than $one hundred and are silent and green enough to run constantly. Make sure the unit you're seeking out is rated HEF'A. HEPA stands for Particulate Air with immoderate overall performance. It is an legitimate smooth out score which means that it captures 0.1 microns (1/a hundredth of a millimeter) and large debris, or ninety nine. Ninety seven percent of airborne stable be counted. So, provide the air within the room an in depth scrubbing, we keep our easy out on low always and run it up for at the least an hour in advance than working within the lab. Finally, to your instantaneous paintings area, you need to clean the air. This can be executed via manner of running internal a glove area, an enclosed space that can be thoroughly disinfected and is draft-free, or in the the front of a go along with the waft hood, a huge HEPA filter out unit that blows a constant waft of herbal sterile air over your workspace, except all contaminants. A glove challenge may be brief and inexpensively set up however is much less powerful because of the truth the air from the distance can discover its manner indoors.

Personal Hygiene

Now that your space has been cleaned and prepared, it is time to consider the opposite primary supply of contamination for your makeshift laboratory: you. Your hair, frame, and garments are an Amazon jungle of bacteria, viruses, and fungi which can be all invisible for your eyes, basically harmless to you or others, however lethal to the mushroom cultures. You have to be as neat as feasible earlier than every art work consultation to hold that nasty horde to a minimal. That technique showering, drying off with a freshly laundered towel and dressing right now in advance than working in a easy set of garments. It's moreover essential to choose out your garb; do no longer put on lengthy-sleeved shirts or free-fitting gadgets that would flop spherical on the equal time as you parent. If you have got were given had been given lengthy hair, tie it up for your head. Use isopropyl (rubbing) alcohol, wash your fingers and lower palms and usually positioned on disposable surgical gloves at the same time as running (wipe the outdoor of the gloves too, use alcohol).

Mental Hygiene

Just as you have got packed your workspace and frame, make certain you're although searching after your country of mind earlier than operating. Mental hygiene is as vital as personal hygiene due to the truth the way you parent might be suffering from your united states of america of mind, and in case you are disturbed or rushed, you are probably to make errors or contaminate your way of lifestyles. Your laboratory moves have to be systematic, calculated and planned. Avoid unnecessary speedy or jerky moves, as they produce handiest undesirable air currents. Take your second. If you're hurried, slow down or hold the idea for a day you have got more time. In the identical way, ask your companion, kids, dog or cat not to go into the room or interrupt you while you're jogging and disconnecting your telephone. Play calming, elevating song in case you need, however avoid Stockhausen or velocity steel, until you find out it in your ears to lighten up.

Chapter 13: Equipment and substances

Mushroom cultivation requires gadget, which includes many unique devices. A couple of these objects are explicit to the point that they have to be provided from mushroom cultivation supply homes, but, maximum can without a whole lot of a stretch be determined at I an series of network assets. A amazing kind of the materials you want fireside likewise offered for a few specific, more and more mundane reason; while making buying much less tough, this has the greater advantage of giving right unfold to those, wishing to live below the radar on their cultivation sports. Home development stores, kitchen, and café supply houses, pup stores, home fermenting organizations, and lawn focuses are the fortune troves of the stealthy (or in truth low priced) mushroom cultivator. Whenever capacity, we've got had been given tried to offer numerous stylish assets to each one of the gadgets you can require.

Equipment

Pressure Cooker

This can be one of the most implemented devices in your cultivation system shed, so it's far important to get a higher than common one proper from the begin. Since you will use it to disinfect usually large gadgets, and in amount, length is easy. If you can control the price of a bigger unit than you earlier than the whole thing want, get it, for the reason that you can probable need to replace later except. The key determinant for what size you have to get is the amount of quart jars you can securely easy right away. Since bricklayer jars are unpredictably authentic, generally few can healthy without trouble internal even the largest pressure cooker, constraining the degree of material you may method right away. In this manner, we propose getting a unit that can hold at least seven-quart jars with out a second's eliminate; the model we use, the All American #941, holds more than two times that many.

There are numerous options as to what brand and type to get, however one stands aside from the group: The All-American logo, synthetic through the Aluminum Foundry of Wisconsin. All American pressure cookers are the wonderful-made, typically dependable, and available to the most strong. The business agency has been doing industrial employer for a long term, and due to the truth that they had been first introduced, the design of their pressure cookers has not basically modified. They're made in famous of overwhelming take a look at forged aluminum, and they do not have elastic seals or placed on-out sections. Replacement additives are conveniently on hand, or maybe a 20-three hundred and sixty five days-vintage unit offered at a secondhand preserve or on eBay may be made to paintings nicely as new.

Like smaller, decrease-priced kitchen pressure cookers, all Americans have a huge, extraordinarily accurate dial scale that lacks a manner of figuring out the inner pressure decisively. They also are purported to hold a vacuum after cooling which is essential to prevent the existence of non-sterile air for your flora.

There are fashionable types of pressure cookers to pick from: people with or similar to a vapor discharge valve, and those with a steel-weighted "rocker" that releases steam at any point above a sure stress degree. The final kind have to be avoided, if possible, as this fast arrival of pressure could likely motive the fluids within the cooker to boil over, dramatically demolishing the media and wrecking. Pressure cookers can be used in rocker fashion, however they want increasingly rigorous monitoring in the course of use to avoid the ones injuries. (Each American makes the 2 types; the kind of stopcock they call strain "sterilizers," on the same time as the weighted rockers are referred to as pressure "canners.") Whatever brand and version of pressure cooker you select out, ensure it's miles in top running order and you recognize its operation and nicely-being (i.E., study the manual). Make exceptional all seals and gaskets match like a play around, and the quilt bolts to the frame tightly. There need to be no steam escaping throughout the seals once it's miles pressurized. Turn off the warm temperature deliver, permit the cooker to calm down absolutely, and nicely reseat the pinnacle if there may be one. Running a Vaseline dot round the threshold of cookers in metal-on-steel layout will make sure an incredible wholesome and assist protect the duvet from seizure to base at some point of use. Before each utilization ensure you add a suitable diploma of water to the bottom of the cooker, anyhow, exact enough to supply the intensity to 1/2 of inch. Never role devices right now at the lowest of the stress cooker, or allow them to touch the outer dividers, in which temperatures are maximum.

Most stress cookers are supported by using way of a rack or trivet presupposed to keep the contents over the water floor and the bigger All-American fashions have basket-customary liners to save you products from direct touch with the cooker itself. Let the stress cooker slowly start to come up to temperature. Excessively quick or lopsided heating can reason packing containers to burst or crack. Until very last the stopcock, constantly convey the cooker to a complete head of steam to displace cooler air wallet. That may additionally take a second, especially on larger cookers. Before shutting the door, you have to see a strong flux of steam coming from the stopcock tube. Never go away unattended an underneath-pressure cooker. The pressure and temperature internal a cooker can change unpredictably, specially at some level within the initial heating intervals, in advance than the cooker even though does now not seem like leveling honestly. It is important that the cooker stay on the right pressure for the entire cycle that permits you to save you a blast and assure complete sanitization. Check it at ordinary intervals or so you can make certain it is not underneath-or overheating and range the source of warmth. Just allow the cooker to kick back slowly and all via itself. Never touch the out of doors of the cooker on the equal time as pressurized, and do not use cold water to chill it even quicker. This can cause the cooker to implode and its contents to discharge savagely. It will generate a large measure of risky electricity, at any charge.

Wrap an alcohol-splashed paper towel around the valve in advance than venting it to release any residual stress to save you unsterile air from being drawn into the strain cooker upon starting. Pressure cookers are probably volatile topics. They produce excessive temperatures and vapor that may purpose harm. Like a very sharp blade, a strain cooker is an machine that needs interest and alertness and therefore offers a terrific advantage.

Petri Dishes

Petri dishes are shallow, transparent plastic or glass dishes with a saggy unfold. They arrive in quite a few sizes, however the most beneficial length for parasitic cultures is 100 x 15 mm. Reusable glass or Pyrex dishes are lengthy enduring and autoclavable but are usually steeply-priced. Pre-sterilized dispensable polystyrene dishes are to be had sleeves of 20 or 25. They are practical, but thinking about that they're presupposed to be used surely once and in some time discarded, they are not actually earth cordial. The types of Petri dishes can be re-sterilized utilizing hydrogen peroxide and a microwave:

1. Wash the plates altogether with dishwashing purifier, taking specific care to totally expel any residual agar.

2. Pour a small degree of 3% peroxide into every dish and whirl it spherical to open it to the entire interior ground of the plate. Repeat with its spread and vicinity it on the dish.

3. Put the pile of dishes in the microwave and warmth at medium stress until all the peroxide has been powered off at the plates.

4. Immediately use the plates or place them in a splendid plastic bag until appropriate.

This technique is preferably paired with the use of peroxide in cultivations of agar. Use pre-sterilized plastic or autoclaved glass dishes is safer while operating with agar which lacks peroxide. We propose the addition of hydrogen peroxide for your cultures at any element practicable to reduce sullying and will will let you art work with agar in a not exactly first-rate circumstance.

In any case, peroxide, for example, cannot be utilized particularly instances whilst generating spores. In those instances, we discover that plaques with a diameter of fifty mm are less complex to preserve clean, due to their decreased surface location. You can use 4-ounce jam jars or similar heatproof glass packing containers if the Petri dishes are unavailable. They have the benefit to be reusable however lack clean lids and absorb extra than two instances as an awful lot area as plates for the network.

Media Flasks

Media flasks are used for containing fluid media at some stage in sanitization and pouring Petri plates. Any thick-walled, autoclavable glass jug will do, but, try to discover one with a usually restricted neck to inspire pouring. One and a half of of-liter squeezed apple or shimmering water bottles with screw pinnacle caps are notable due to this.

Mason Jars

We use fantastic Ball-fashion mason canning jars, usually in quart sizes. They are without troubles reachable, strong, and may be reused uncertainly. For grain spawn, constrained mouth (70 mm) quart jars are nice. In the occasion that you need to try the so-referred to as "PF" method, you will need proper away-sided, half of of-sixteen oz. Jam jars.

A study of alert: mason jars are strong; however, they do from time to time damage. Always evaluate them closely in advance than use for cracks, dispose of suspicious-looking ones straight away, and be more careful whilst shaking jars of grain. Don't smack them down onto the palm of your hand to split the grains; a cracked jar can take a finger right away off. Instead, actually keep the jar via the lid give up and shake it right proper right here and there. In the event that the grain is absolutely firmly fine, and also you want to ruin it up persuasively, cautiously hit the jar in the route of a spotless towel supported thru a thick cushion or closer to a halfway used float of pipe tape till it slackens up. (Make first rate that the lid is firmly constant too; you do not need your precious spawn flying all over the region.) Always allow your strain cooker to warmth up often; speedy heating can purpose jars to crack due to the temperature distinction among their insides and outsides.

Mason Jar Lids

Don't mess with the metal lids given in portions; spare the ones for canned tomatoes. We use a one-piece plastic lid for culture paintings, this is heat-resistant and modified with out problems to allow the criminal alternate of gasoline. The ball makes a "Stockpiling Cap" plastic. Even despite the fact that the bundling notes that those caps are "not for garage," they're sincerely autoclavable. You will carefully bore or lessen an I-inch hole inside the focal element of every cap to modify the ones lids. When prepared with a filter out circle (see subsequent section), the ones modified caps allow gasses (now not however contaminants) to undergo the jar during, so that your cultures can breathe freely.

Filter Disks

Placed between the lid and the jar's mouth, clear out plates permit the trade of gases with out contaminants being uncovered. They are made from a warmth resistant artificial fiber and can be often sterilized.

They are multiple millimeters thick and come pre-lessen to fit the proper jar-and-lid combo. Occasionally, at the identical time as in touch with soil or shape spores, they discolor. In that case, clearly drill them on a medium-time period foundation in a 1/four-wonderful fade affiliation (i.E., 1/4-CUP standard first rate dye in three/4-Cup water) not like the ones plates, an low value possibility is Tyvek, which can be lessen to in shape over the jar lid. Tyvek is a synthetic cloth that is applied in pretty a variety of programs.

Building deliver shops will buy rolls, and smaller portions are to be had to Ups or the U.S. For not anything. Mail station like the ones oversized, indestructible envelopes for mailing. Beca the use of Tyvek is thinner and extra bendy than the company filter out plates, it need to be reduce extra deeply round and spherical than the jarhead, and one inch will preserve off the threshold of the jar. Tyvek is likewise reusable however ought to be discarded after 3 or 4 packages.

Spawn Bags

Otherwise known as clean out repair baggage, those are apparent, warmth-resistant, gusseted flexible plastic baggage used to maintain large spawning quantities. They are autoclavable and characteristic on one detail a small square filter out for changing air. They are stacked with soil, sterilized, immunized, and glued with an impulse (warm temperature) sealer afterward. They are appropriate for growing out huge quantities of spawn due to the fact they're versatile, and it is possible to control or analyze the interior contents for pollutants with out try. They lose their heating versatility and are generally accurate for solitary use best, but baggage in shape as a mess around may be in truth cleaned out and sterilized all once more.

We've visible farmers use "oven luggage" (or spawns) within the grocery save. While these are autoclavable and may be made to paintings, they lack a clean out restore that does not exactly offer an top notch alternate of gas, and they will be too small to even consider seal heating. One way to equip this type of bag with a few breathability is to wrap its neck tightly spherical a thick wad of polyfill or cotton and seal it firmly with a considerable breathability

Impulse Sealer

Impulse sealers are used for solving spawn bags. Make sure to get one large sufficient to straddle the entire bag on the identical time as extended flat, at any fee, 12 inches throughout. E-Bay is a wonderful vicinity to search for gives on impulse sealers.

Alcohol Lamp

This is a tumbler lamp with a cotton wick and metallic neckline. Loaded up with scouring alcohol, it offers a spotless hearth to disinfecting surgical gadget and inoculation loops as you determine.

Then over again, you may use a:

Mini torch

Sold in kitchen deliver homes for caramelizing the outdoor layer on creme Brule, and bought in devices stores for soldering, those smaller than traditional butane lighting fixtures are beneficial for disinfecting gear as you work. A unique wonderful one can have a strong base to keep it upstanding even as it sits at the seat top.

Balance

Mechanical or virtual models are further outstanding. The vital traits to look for in a stability are precision to in any event 0.Five g, the capability to weigh as a whole lot as at least 250 g (1 kg is better) and a dish sufficiently massive to healthy outsized gadgets.

Surgical blade

Surgical blades are used for reducing and moving agar and tissue cultures. A skinny-handled dismembering surgical tool with dispensable #10-sized sharp edges is right. If you can't discover the ones, an all-aluminum Xacto-style blade will artwork OK, however, it has an inclination to be to a few diploma more tough to transport into tight regions.

Inoculation Loop

This wire loop toward the give up of a metallic or wood deal with is used to move spores or small measures of mycelium to agar plates. It very well may be found in logical or brew making deliver shops or made from a dowel and a chunk of skinny robust wire. An inoculation loop isn't always required within the occasion which you use the "cardboard circle" method of spore germination.

Sharpies

This perpetual compose anywhere markers are important for naming culture packing containers of all kind.

Pipes

It is useful to have varieties of plastic or steel channels: a thin necked one for pouring fluids and extremely good powders, and a massive-mouthed one for filling jars.

Estimating [Serological) Pipette and Rubber Bulb

If you need to paintings with agar, you may need some way of estimating small volumes of fluid (1-15 mL) to add in your cultures. Ten-milliliter glass estimating pipettes are pleasant because of this considering that they're autoclavable, reusable, and function markings on them to effortlessly determine volume. An elastic bulb is used to draw and administer fluids from the pipette. Both may be determined at logical vendors and some domestic combination stores. A glass 10-milliliter graduated chamber or a set of steel estimating spoons can be used for that reason, however, it's going to require even extra handling and care to keep away from polluting your cultures at the identical time as you determine.

Graduated Cylinders

These are used to efficiently quantify fluids. Cylinders in l-liter, 1 OO-milliliter, and 10-milliliter sizes ought to recall every contingency.

Measuring cups and spoons

Measuring cups and spoons may be utilized in location of graduated tubes however are much less specific to three diploma. For l-cup (250rnl) to 8-cup (2 L) numbers, use Pyrex ones, and for smaller quantities use metallic ones. Where sterility is needed in advance than use, the 2 kinds may be autoclaved or sterilized in boiling water (5 minutes at a moving boil).

Syringes

Syringes are used to do mass inoculation in spore, a machine referred to as "Psilocybe Fanaticus." Ten-or twenty-milliliter sizes are used, which include large bore needles (18-degree). In a strain cooker, they may be autoclaved times, or sterilized in boiling water. From careful and veterinary retail shops, and from a few on-line providers of mushroom factors, syringes can be offered.

In any event, their settlement is regulated in severa U.S. States, and that they can be elusive locally at instances. When you purchase spore syringes pre-filled, after use, smooth and spare the syringe and needle. They are autoclavable and generally reusable.

Supplies

Hydrogen Peroxide (3%)

This antiseptic is added to cultures to shield them from defilement. It is obtainable at most pharmacies or grocery shops. The actual convergence of hydrogen peroxide arrangements every so often fluctuates, so make certain the date at the bottle is of overdue vintage (See sidebar under for a way of locating hydrogen peroxide's attention level). Right now, is generally innocent to human fitness and requires no particular coping with strategies, besides wearing gloves. It is a mellow fading operator, so be cautious not to dribble it onto garb.

Increasingly centered (8-35%) arrangements are available from an entire lot of assets, for example, pool supply shops, and at the net. Hydrogen peroxide in focuses greater than three% can reason intense consumes and is probably flamable, so be cautious even as working with it. Peroxide corrupts quite brief, to protect that it remains at the proper attention, use the bottle at the earliest possibility next to commencing. Between makes use of, envelop the neck and cap with the useful useful resource of parafilm or plastic wrap, and save the bottle interior a spotless plastic bag within the cooler. Prior to each use, wipe down the out of doors of the bottle and cap (counting the mouth and neck beneath the cap) with alcohol, and take uncommon care no longer to touch any piece of the bottle itself collectively with your palms or device on the equal time as apportioning. Always sanitize pipettes and graduated cylinders as a manner to come into touch with peroxide earlier than use, both in a strain cooker alongside facet your media or thru submerging them in boiling water for five mins.

Isopropyl [Rubbing) Alcohol

This is used for sanitizing palms, surfaces and containers, and as gasoline for alcohol lamps. It is offered in grocery shops and pharmacies in each 70% or 91 % focuses, every of it is low price. Cautioning: Isopropanol is profoundly flamable!! Get it far from open blazes, if you do not thoughts make certain some thing alcohol you have got got used has virtually evaporated earlier than you moderate your alcohol lamp.

Blanch

Standard wonderful laundry dye is beneficial for cleaning surfaces and equipment. Avoid producers with introduced cleansers. Weaken to in any occasion 1/4 extremely good in advance than use. A 10% pleasant arrangement in a sprig bottle is an awesome ground and air disinfectant.

Parafilm

Parafilm is a paraffin-based totally absolutely in reality, flexible film carried out to seal Petri dishes. It is gas permeable, which means that that that it takes below attention gasoline alternate even as keeping contaminants out of cultures. An tremendous shape in 1-inchwide rolls is sold by means of manner of way of some lawn deliver corporations as "Uniting Tape." If you can't find out Parafilm, you may opportunity polyethylene stick movie, as an instance, Glad Wrap (but no longer Saran Wrap or comparable producers, which can be made from polyvinylchloride and are not gasoline permeable.). Utilizing a pointy blade, cautiously lessen a 1-to 2-inch-big phase off the end of a whole roll.

Surgical Gloves

Dispensable latex gloves are critical for buying grimy arms a protracted way out of your best cultures. They need not be pre-sterilized. Simply wash your fingers and fingers a long time earlier than placing them on, at that aspect wipe the outdoor of the gloves with an alcohol-soaking moist paper towel (commonly allow them to dry truly earlier than going anyplace near an open fireplace.)

Substrates & Casing Materials

Whole Grains

For spawn creation, the most usually used substrate is entire grain. Entire grains make a fantastic mechanism for spawn for some of motives. Each grain demonstrations like a smaller than normal tablet of nutritional nutritional dietary supplements, minerals, and water that is handily colonized via the usage of higher fungi, on the same time as its sinewy husk halfway shields it from infection with the aid of way of special dwelling beings. Upon colonization, the grains are efficaciously separated from every precise. At prolonged last, at the same time as colonized grain spawn is used to immunize mass substrates, every grain fills in at least vicinity of mycelium and supplement holds, a miles flung station from which the fungus can soar off onto the contemporary medium.

While almost any cereal grain will artwork as spawn, we suggest sensitive wintry weather (white) wheat, as it has labored properly for us, and is by using the use of all bills liberated from the bacterial contaminants that can be present on rye and specific grains. You may additionally moreover use some thing grains are pretty sincerely available to u, however we do advocate the usage of massive bit grains like rye, wheat, or corn, rather than small-grained cereals like millet or rice, which have a tendency to cluster together while cooked. We have seen some growers use wild birdseed combination with well results, which has the easy little little little bit of leeway of being modest and genuinely handy. Be that as it could, due to the reality it's miles a mixture of severa sized grains, birdseed is increasingly more hard to moisten because it have to be. It can likewise be very clingy whilst damp. To limit those problems, hydrate birdseed with a 24-hour cold soak in location of boiling water, and flush and drain it thoroughly earlier than stacking into bins. You need to attempt to use natural grains at some factor element workable, for the purpose that this is the wonderful manner to assure that they have now not been handled with fungicides.

Malt Extract, Dried

This is a powdered extract of grains which have been "malted" or superior to expand the unfinished transformation of their starch into sugars. Malt extract is used as an essential alternative in agar merchandise. It is consequences accessible from getting prepared vendors. Make advantageous to use slight or tan malt. Darker malts have been caramelized and fungi are not growing properly on caramelized sugars.

Yeast Extract

A dried extract of yeast cells, plentiful in vitamins, minerals, and protein, yeast extract is added to agar media as a healthful enhancement. Brewer's yeast, handy in severa fitness meals shops, is an good sufficient opportunity, however it isn't always as effective as evident yeast extract.

Calcium Carbonate [CaC03)

Calcium carbonate is otherwise referred to as lime, hydrated lime, limestone flour, clam shell flour, and chalk. It is used to cradle the pH of packaging soils and substrates, demoralize contamination, and offer calcium to the growing fungus. Fungi generally generally tend to select barely essential (as an instance pH > 8) media, at the same time as microbes and a few wonderful contaminants do no longer. Check the selection to make certain the calcium carbonate you purchase is low in magnesium « 1 %), due to the fact a few fungi do not increase properly on substrates containing excessive measures of it.

Calcium Sulfate

Also referred to as gypsum, calcium sulfate is used to capture overabundance water in substrates, making them less difficult to shake or separate, and assisting with preventing water logging and infection. It is essentially impartial in pH and has no buffering functionality.

Hardwood Sawdust and Chips

These are substrates for the genus Psilocybe cyanescens, P. Azurescens and related lignicolous species (timber-owning). Birch, cottonwood, oak, birch, and beech are appropriate, despite the fact that maximum hardwood species will do so. In case you have got got any of these tree species growing close by, you can have the selection to get sparkling chips from your close by highway administrative center or lawn popularity, in any other case you might be able to chip your private. Chips superior in wintry weather or late wintry climate from timber are first-class as they will be maximum in sugars and encompass at least inexperienced count number number variety, which can be a contamination vector in beds.

You can from time to time get close by hardwood chips from grill vendors, who marketplace them for use in meals smokers. If you do now not address hardwoods regionally, you can purchase wood chips online. Fine chipped wood beech or maple chips are marketed as creature bedding (Beta-Chip and SaniChip are manufacturers to pay particular hobby to), however they're generally too first rate to even suggest the usage of on my own, and want to be paired with large chips or a few element to have an impact on them.

Sawdust Fuel Pellets

Used for domestic heating in particular timber stoves, those are crafted from sawdust compressed into tiny pellets. During manufacturing, the excessive heat generated: makes them quite sterile. The pellets fall into sawdust another time while they are moistened with warmness water. This item is to be had at domestic heating providers similarly to 3 home improvement shops. Stove pellets make a excellent supply of sawdust for substrates-clearly make sure to get a logo made from hardwoods best. In some of tree species, along with birch and oak, they're furthermore sold as fuel to food individuals who smoke.

Spiral-Grooved Dowels

Spiral-grooved dowels are resultseasily to be had from woodworking carriers as fixtures-turning into a member of pegs; the incredible ones for mushroom use are 1 to two inches long and 1/4-inch or five/16-inch in diameter. They are usually crafted from birch and may be assigned thusly. They are maximum generally applied in mushroom cultivation on logs, in which the colonized pegs are beat into openings throughout the perimeter of the log. The spiral furrow around the out of doors of the peg offers a maximal floor place from which the mycelium can jump off onto resulting substrates.

Paper Pellet Cat Litter

Used for the capacity of cultures in small glass tubes. The free, open form and constrained nourishing content material material of paper makes it best for the prolonged-term protection of most mushroom species. Search for a logo that is unscented and product of 100% reused paper; Crown, Good Mews, and Yesterday's News are three brands we've got were given decided to be effective.

Peat Moss

A factor of casing soil, peat moss is sold in lawn focuses everywhere in the location. While it has minimum wholesome gain, its excessive-water retaining capability gives dampness to the growing fruitbodies. It is to a few degree acidic and need to be cradled with calcium carbonate.

Vermiculite

Vermiculite is every other element of casing soil. It is used for its water preserving capability, and its easy, open structure, which allows appropriate gasoline change. It is offered at many garden agencies. Use the coarsest grade you can discover. There is a delusion that vermiculite includes asbestos, which isn't valid. Apparently, there has been a solitary vermiculite mine in Montana that modified into debased with asbestos, and it have become closed. After this episode became post moss and vermiculite. Different manufacturers started attempting out their vermiculite for asbestos, but it changed into no longer decided anywhere else. In any case, vermiculite and similar substances (like peat and calcium salts) do contain a super deal of extremely notable particulates, which may be risky every time breathed in. Always placed on a painter's residue veil even as dealing with them in their dry united states of america.

Chapter 14: PF TEK Improved

In this bankruptcy, along side our refinements of it, we describe the well-known "Psilocybe Fanaticus" mushroom cultivation approach, otherwise called the "PF Tek." This approach is the primary tool to be uncovered to for masses Psilocybe mushroom growers these days, so we felt it modified into crucial that we cover it in our e-book, notwithstanding the reality that we do no longer understand it as a latest exercise. Since it's far as just like foolproof as a technique of growing mushrooms can get, it's miles a wonderful place to start for a amateur. It requires a minimal investment of time and value, and in a rather short time exposes the beginner to the whole lifestyles cycle of a mushroom. Taking a near and number one-hand look at this method will will assist you to recognize the thoughts that underlie the more complicated strategies that comply with. If you pick out to begin your mushroom cultivation with a Psilocybe cubensis spore-water syringe in preference to a spore print, this approach is a incredible way to use it (notwithstanding the truth that now not the quality one: you can also use it to right away inoculate grain spawning. The method lets in you to proper away produce a natural fruiting pressure of P. Cubensis, with minimum interference. Above this is located a skinny layer of dry vermiculite, found via some layers of aluminum foil. The brown rice flour offers the colonization of the fungus with a wholesome nutrient base, at the same time as the vermiculite acts as a reservoir for water and lets in create an open, ethereal form that allows the developing vegetation to respire. The jars are then sterilized in a strain cooker or bath with boiling water. Upon cooling, the primary layer of foil is removed, and at various points throughout the jar's diameter the jars are without problems whole of some milliliters of a spore solution from a syringe. The top layer of foil is changed, and the jars are then located in an incubator or a heat, draft-unfastened spot. With time the spores will germinate and fuse to shape a dikaryotic mycelium with an appropriate mate.

In each injection, the big form of spores ensures that mating will rise up and that each jar contains a large type of traces. The many traces present are competing to colonize the jar, with the weaker ones being overtaken through the most whole of existence (and by way of using extension, maximum likely to well undergo fruit). The jars should be simply colonized after some weeks or so and are prepared to be fruited. The "cakes" of mycelium are knocked out of the jars at this element inside the genuine PF Tek and positioned the incorrect way up on a bed of moistened perlite at the bottom of a easy box collectively with an aquarium or a plastic garage bin, this is protected to preserve immoderate humidity stages. The fruiting chamber is located beneath a slight supply (fluorescent lighting fixtures develop associated with a timer or possibly a brightly illuminated window). Once or instances a day, the duvet is removed, and the desserts are fanned via hand to get rid of built-up CO_2, then misted with water from a hand spray bottle. In time, primordia form on the cake's outer floor and ultimately ripen into complete-sized mushrooms. We go away the substratum in the jar in our "progressed" PF Tek, and mushrooms fruit best from the top surface of the jar. This serves a chain of ends. One, it receives rid of the need for perlite tubs that are tough and messy. Instead, the jars are perforated into any clean enclosed box, or perhaps a plastic bag, to permit alternate of gasoline.

Second, the want for excessive ambient humidity is decreased, due to the fact the top layer of herbal vermiculite acts as a casing layer, preserving a reservoir of water that may be drawn from the growing give up stop result. Because fruiting is confined to a horizontal floor, the forming mushrooms keep a far extra herbal look and form. On the opposite hand, the proper "cake" method tends to deliver stop cease end result of peculiar patterns and sizes, as they develop throughout the cake at random elements. (Since spores are maximum successfully dispersed from downward-handling gills, most mushrooms employ gravity to orient themselves horizontally. If, as in our approach, the stipes are already pointing inside the proper path, they manifestly broaden right away and tall.) By incorporating a casing layer, the "improved" PF Tek resembles extra cautiously the advanced strategies that we later gift. You'll be extra than familiar with the essential mushroom lifestyles cycle after you have got achieved this technique a couple of instances, and prepared to transport on.

The "Improved" PF Tek

Materials forty mL (meager '/4 cup) natural brown rice flour (regular with jar) a hundred and forty mL ('/2 cup) vermiculite (in line with jar), in addition to extra for casing layer

Water half of of of-sixteen ounces. (250 mL) mason jars Aluminum foil Spore-water syringe(s)

Alcohol lamp or butane lighter Rubbing alcohol

Material Notes: Brown rice flour is obtainable at a few health food shops, or you can pound your private in a touch espresso processor or zest manufacturing unit. The jars should be immediately sided Gelly jars), with out the shoulders present on big-sized canning jars. Faucet water is brilliant; however, you can use bottled or delicate in case your water deliver is suspect.

Sterilization Note: This method includes the only prevalence right now we depict a boiling water shower cleansing of a substrate as a choice to pressure-cooking.

The water shower method is strong, however now not 1 00% dependable; a few percentage of jars prepared with it will at present be in all likelihood to taint. In the event that you have a stress cooker, you want to use it proper right here as well; if now not, presently is as appropriate a time as any to get one.

1.   Depending on the kind of jars you may vaccinate (a 10 mL syringe includes sufficient solution for immunize 8-10 jars), vicinity the important degree of vermiculite in a bowl. Presently evacuate around 5% of this and place it in a separate problem.

2.   Into the precept bowl of vermiculite, upload water a piece at a time, blending as you skip, till the mixture can't maintain any longer and tl1ere is pleasant a mild overabundance of water at the bottom of the bowl. Presently upload the held dry fabric and mix certainly. The vermiculite need to now be at "discipline capacity," implying that it includes the most excessive

degree of water it is able to without issue preserve.

three.	Empty the brown rice flour into the bowl and blend nicely, masking the vermiculite grains with a layer of moistened flour.

4.	Spoon this combination into the jars, leaving a diploma half-inch (1-centimeter) hole on the pinnacle. Place it into the jars freely and do no longer percentage it down; maintaining an open, breezy shape will allow the mycelium to breath and expand at a awesome price. Take a clammy paper towel and wipe down the edges and round internal edges of the jars to sincerely expel any wanderer substrate, that might in a few manner trade right into a deliver of infection.

five.	Occupy the relaxation of the space of the jar with dry vermiculite. This layer will earlier than the entirety pass about as a quandary to contaminants, which, need to they through one way or a few other discover their way within the jar, would be averted from stepping into contact with the substrate. Afterward, it'll fill in because of the reality the casing soil, from which the mushrooms will fruit.

6.   Take five-inch square bits of aluminum foil and wrap them firmly over the mouth of the jar. Freely screw lids onto the jars, taking care not to rip the foil underneath. (The use of lids within the PF Tek is discretionary however presents an additional layer of guarantee.)

7.   Burden the jars into your pressure cooker, on the facet of the right degree of water, and sanitize the jars at 15 psi for forty five minutes. If there is enough room, the jars is probably stacked in more than one layer.

Or then again (Boiling Water Bath Method):

8.   Place the jars in a big cooking pot in a solitary layer, alongside facet enough water

to deliver it to about midway up the rims of the jars. Spread the pot and boil for 1 .Five hours. Check every now and then to ensure the water diploma remains constant, which includes water as crucial.

Phase 2: PF Tek Inoculation

1.   When the jars have cooled proper proper right down to room temperature, located them on a smooth working floor, together with the spore-water syringe and alcohol lamp. Replace the lids and drop the cover over the pinnacle foil.

2.   Remove the duvet from the syringe, rub the needle with a moistened alcohol, smooth paper towel or cotton ball, and area the pinnacle of the needle for your lamp's flame until it starts offevolved glowing red (be cautious to maintain the plastic cease of the needle a long way from the flame, and be cautious on the equal time as using alcohol close to an open flame).

3.   Using one container at a time, removing the pinnacle layer of tape, shaking the syringe lightly to disperse the spore solution, and injecting a small quantity into the jar at four similarly spaced dots proper within the internal rim. Insert 1 inch (2 cm) of needle into the jar so its factor passes the dry layer of vermiculite, then squeeze out some drops. You need to be in a niche to look the answer run down the jar sides. Repeat on 3 factors left. Every jar should get 1-1, 5 mL normal solution.

4.   Inject all the jars within the identical manner, shielding the top layer of foil and cap (if used) at every. Label the outdoor of the jars with relevant information and/or pocket e book range, and role in a smooth, heat spot to incubate.

Phase 3: Incubation

The jars must be incubated in the seventy five-850 F variety, at a warm, draft-unfastened vicinity. If your property temperature is continuously interior this range, then it have to be enough to in reality store them in a clean problem. If no longer, an incubator box will make certain healthful and speedy growth, and is simple to assemble from a cooler and some devices that you could purchase from a domestic dog shop's reptile branch.

Materials

☐   25-50 gallon plastic or Styrofoam cooler

☐   8 watt reptile heating mat

☐   Flexible indoor regulator controller

☐   Air temperature thermometer

Place the heating mat and thermometer inside the cooler, plug the mat in and turn on the temperature controller. Set the controller to its lowest placing and allow the cooler warmth up for a few hours in advance than switching it up step by step until it reaches a regular eighty ° or some thing like this. Arrange the heating mat on one side of the cooler, and stack your jars at the alternative facet, as an prolonged manner from direct heat as might be allowed. Depending on the surrounding temperature of the room, you could need to via the way alter the indoor regulator to hold a consistent temperature inside the cooler. At the issue at the identical time as surrounding temperatures cross above 80 5°, you'll need to make experience of a way to shield the jars from overheating. Right now, then developing an complex refrigeration tool, your most logical choice is to keep them in a near box in a groovy spot in your own home, as an example, an unheated basement. If no such place is offered to you, this would be a great time to take a destroy for a while, until out of doors temperatures have cooled properly to hold cultivation.

Phase 4: Germination/Colonization

Within consistent with week or so, the primary signs and symptoms of spore germination on your jars will start to seem. Look for tiny pinpoints of fantastic white fozzy boom, generally right away below the injection points near the lowest of the jar. Those tiny colonies radiate outward in time to form character mycelium spheres. The spheres interior each jar can be part of every distinct interior 10 days to three weeks, and the jar can be absolutely colonized.

Contamination

The jar is in all likelihood to be infected in case you see any boom on your jars that isn't herbal white in colour and need to be removed from the incubator right now and disposed of. Molds which have a tendency to have specially coloured spores in sun shades of blue, green, black or crimson is probably the most not unusual offenders. On the other hand, bacterial contamination will appear as spots of wet, sticky blobs at the jar's internal ground, and can be discovered with the beneficial resource of a bitter or rotten smell of apples. Remember to generally do away with infected tradition containers from your paintings and developing regions, and thoroughly easy the bins earlier than returning them to your workspace.

Phase five: Fruiting

Once the jars have colonized simply, they will be prepared to be fruited. At this diploma, the lids and foil are removed, the top layer of vermiculite is moistened, and the jars are placed underneath a moderate deliver, either thru artificial moderate given via a dedicated fluorescent "increase" light or by using a brightly lit window. Since P cubensis requires light to stimulate fruiting, and you need to restriction fruiting to the pinnacle surface of the desserts, you want to restrict mild exposure to really that place of the jars in some way. This can be finished in severa numbers of methods, together with wrapping the jars in aluminum foil, or thick, opaque paper strips. One simple method that we used is to vicinity the jars internal short quantities of cardboard tubing, collectively with the sort used to save posters, reduce to go back back just above the rim.

Preparing the Jars for Fruiting

1.   Remove the lids and foil from each jar. You may see a few "fans" of mycelium jabbing up thru the vermiculite layer.

2.   Wipe a spotless fork with a few alcohol, allow it to evaporate, and in some time delicately scratch (not scratch off) the dry vermiculite layer right all the manner all the way down to the top of the cake beneath, to break up and equitably flow into the mycelial elements internal.

3.   Take a twig mister of smooth water and mist the vermiculite till it's miles saturated (it'll darken slightly in coloration; at the same time as you can see unfastened streaming water, that is enough.)

4.   Repeat with each jar, cleaning the fork each time to save you inadvertently spreading contaminants.

5.   At the element at the same time as everything of the jars is prepared, place them in singular cardboard cylinders interior an encased field, as an instance, a massive easy plastic bag (reduce or perforate it to provide a few fuel alternate) or an cheaper plastic stockpiling bathtub.

6.   If you're using a fluorescent grow moderate, set your timer to an 8-hour on 1 sixteen-hour off cycle; in any case, genuinely discover the jars in a sufficiently vibrant region, as an example, close to a radiant window. The fine temperature of your growing location need to be within the sixty five-75°F variety, barely lower than that required throughout colonization.

7.   Mist the casing gently a few instances every day to replace any water lost to vanishing.

You have to see primordia begin to shape inside multiple days to approximately fourteen days. They will no doubt grow in the casing layer and will not be seen till small-scale mushrooms are already mounted all round. They will be predisposed to develop astonishingly rapid once they have completed this scale and may seem to attain at whole period honestly medium time period. They will draw water from the cake and the casing layer as they amplify, so make certain to growth misting severa to preserve the vermiculite saturated, usually taking care no longer to overwater.

Phase 6: Harvesting at the same time as the mushroom has reached a appropriate length for a success spore dispersal, it stops growing and will growth its cap to reveal the surroundings to its spore-providing gills. This argument is best accompanied via the pleasant time to pick your mushrooms, as a unmarried mushroom can launch a galactic amount of spores, that could make topics pretty chaotic. When the mushroom prepares to expose its gills the remarkable way to tell is to pay close to interest to the partial veil, the skinny protective film that covers them. At first, at the same time as the cap is virtually inserted (searching lots like the ones relevant vintage streetlamps globe-on - a-shaft), the partial veil is blanketed up). As the cap starts to boom, the veil workplace paintings throughout the cap's backside hemisphere as a spherical, moderate-coloured band.

When the cap begins offevolved to flatten out, the partial veil receives extended beyond its capacity to expand and begins to tear, pulling away from the external edges of the gills. Eventually, the partial veil withdraws from the cap altogether, and its remainders live joined to the stipe in a skirt-like ring, known as an annulus). Ideally, you want to pick out your mushrooms at the same time as the partial veil is visible, or at the most current, earlier than it starts offevolved to interrupt. Harvesting the mushrooms is as primary as getting a cope with on them at the bottom and winding tenderly on the identical time as pulling them an extended way up into the clouds from the casing. In the occasion that your palms are small and deft sufficient, you could use your spotless fingers to do as such; if no longer, more than one easy chopsticks makes an awesome harvesting gadget. Any piece of the mushroom that very last components in the back of within the casing will rot, so take care to eliminate the whole lot, right all the way right down to the base of the stipe. Do a few element it takes now not to the touch the casing layer and take uncommon care now not to harm close by less-created mushrooms or primordia. Sometimes, be that as it may, it's miles difficult to keep away from frightening or evacuating nearby mushrooms while expelling some different. Right now, is smarter to dispose of those "babies" also, in desire to leaving them within the lower returned of. Often, frightening them cuts off their association with the substrate and they prevent developing and in the end rot. What energy the manner of life might come what may additionally, or another have expended on those stop stop result can be occupied to one-of-a-kind humans, so do no longer pressure masses over the rare loss.

Normally, a first rate measure of vermiculite is probably adhered to the bottom of the harvested mushrooms, leaving behind a divot within the casing layer. When you're finished harvesting, actually fill the ones holes with easy vermiculite, mist the casing altogether and move again the jars to their fruiting place. During the period proper now following a harvest, increment misting recurrence altogether, so as to update the superb measure of dampness eliminated from the cakes.

Each jar want to produce three to 5 yields, or flushes, of mushrooms, with about seven days of healing time among every harvest.

During the later flushes, whilst the nutritional dietary supplements of the substrate are notably worn-out, the desserts will decrease and shy away from the sides of the jar, uncovering the dividers of the cakes to the surroundings and to slight. Mushrooms will at that problem start to form at some stage in the facets of the desserts. Aside fro111. Being an increasing number of hard to eliminate surely from the jar, the ones aren't an issue (that is the location multiple chopsticks proves to be useful).

After the fourth or fifth flush, the jars is probably almost truly tired, and the amount of mushrooms that shape can be insignificant. Now, the cakes need to be discarded, for the cause that mycelium in them will start to bypass on and will sooner or later rot, becoming a vector for infection.

Chapter 15: Working with agar

Preparing Agar Plates

Mushroom plant life are commonly grown out on nitrified agar plates and maintained. The agar's easy, semi-solid surface offers an outspread, two-dimensional boom pattern, considering the smooth assessment of a crop and the specific proof of and separation from any pollution that want to upward push up. Agar is a polysaccharide (a sugar-like atom) located in the mobile dividers of certain green boom. At the component even as disintegrated in boiling water and in some time cooled, agar partially solidifies, much like gelatin.

Agar itself gives no sustenance to the fungus, so some of dietary supplements are delivered to the medium, for instance, malt sugar and yeast extract. The fixings are mixed with water in a heatproof box, sterilized in a strain cooker, and crammed Petri dishes at the same time as although fluid. One of the media most commonly used is Malt-Yeast Extract Agar, or MYA, for brief. It is a usually useful medium, one on which all species of Psilocybe will broaden gracefully.

Senescence

Growers frequently interchange media recipes to avoid pressure senescence, the corruption of a way of life because of maturing. Sometimes after a number of transfers among plates, a culture can begin to grow feebly, or perhaps prevent developing interior and out. Senescent cultures typically have a tendency to fruit inadequately or now not in the slightest diploma and are typically discarded for re-separation of a healthful strain from spores.

The causes of pressure senescence are however now not simply information; but, it appears to occur frequently whilst a culture is maintained on similar media recipe for an prolonged time-body. Fungi (like people) seem to do first-rate even as given numerous meals to expend, and like us they increase exhausted or even pass on at the same time as given something very just like eat day in, day ride. To keep away from senescence, it is number one which you trade your media recipe every time you operate it, which "works out" the fungus, horrifying it to provide numerous units of proteins constantly. One primary manner to do that is to add small quantities of grain flour to every bunch, rotating the sort you operate each time you pour new plates, as portrayed below. Once in some time, anyhow, you want to project your fungus substantially similarly, with the useful useful resource of requesting that it grow on a very novel medium. This may be specifically beneficial for restoring a way of life that begins offevolved to expose evidence of debilitating. Right now, want to reject every primary sugar and starches clearly, and deliver it some detail completely novel to way. (We call this recipe "Anything" Agar.)

It may want to probably amplify regularly at the modern medium, however following half of a month of boom, on the identical time as you flow into it lower once more to an an increasing number of balanced medium like MYA, it's miles probable to detonate with new boom. What wouldn't it be a remarkable idea on the manner to feed it? Any cellulose, starch, or sugar will do, which encompass soybeans, paper pellets, raspberry jam, nutty spread some issue you might imagine approximately. The sky's the factor of confinement. We have even identified about one cultivator who took care of his fungi dried crickets he determined at a doggy save! Now and over again you may discover a fabric that your fungi refuse to boom on. Assuming that is the case, no problem, really take a stab at a few aspect else. Another manner to avoid strain debasement is to restrict the amount of transfers of every life-style which you carry out.

☐   Malt Yeast Agar [MYA] Medium

☐   22 g agar

☐   12 g light malt extract

☐   1 g yeast extract

☐   1/four tsp natural grain flour (rotate among oats, cornmeal, amaranth, rice, millet, rye or a few distinctive starch or sugar you can hold in mind)

☐   five g wood fuel pellets or hardwood sawdust

☐   1 L tap water 8 mL 3% hydrogen peroxide (discretionary, added after sanitization and cooling; see beneath.)

1.   Add every unmarried dry solving to jar, found by way of the usage of the water. Make sure to use a jar this is 1 .Five to 2 instances the quantity of media favored, so it does now not boil over all through cleansing. Attachment the neck of the bottle with cotton fleece, at that trouble wrap the

hole and neck of the bottle with aluminum foil.

2.   Put the jar inside the strain cooker at the side of the essential diploma of water. If you may add peroxide to the agar, make sure to sterilize some estimating pipettes too, wrapped in aluminum toil to preserve up sterility earlier than use.

three.   Sterilize at 15 psi for 30 min. Try not to put together dinner your agar media for longer than forty five minutes, considering that this could motive the media to caramelize, and fungi do no longer broaden well on caramelized sugars.

four.   Permit the strain cooker to return back to atmospheric pressure, at that element cautiously skip the jar and pipettes to a glove enclose or front of a movement hood while though hot. It is useful to use a few layers of easy paper towel as a potholder while moving objects from the stress cooker to the workspace.

five. When the usage of peroxide: observe eight mL of three percent hydrogen peroxide, the use of a sterile channel e or calculating spoon, till the out of doors of the box is co (' l enough to address speedy but very hot on the identical time (among 1' zero °-a hundred and forty ° F). In the 2 headings, rotate the medium gently a few instances to combination it in altogether. Be careful now not to over-agitate it and construct bubbles that emerge as in your dishes.

6. Open your Petri dishes sleeves as deliberate at the bundling and stack them at once onto your paintings region. To later electricity deliver plastic jacket.

7. Operating with stacks of ten plates one after the alternative, decorate the whole stack thru the lid of the lowest plate in a unmarried hand, leaving the bottom half of on the pinnacle of the table, and slowly sell off absolutely enough medium into the plate to definitely cover it. Replace the

stack, and repeat until entire, with the plate above. One liter of common will suffice for everyday Petri dishes of 20-30 1 00 mm. Make an attempt no longer to agitate while you pour within the combination. When strong particles are at the lowest of the cup, go away them there; all usable vitamins must be in affiliation, and you need the media for your plates to be obvious sufficient to look via.

eight.   If you locate that the agar begins to solidify in advance than you end pouring it, protective the jar in a shallow pot of warm (1 50 ° F) water while now not being used is frequently beneficial.

9.   Stack the finished plates in a single section, and freely replace the sleeve they got here in to permit every plate inside the stack to sit back grade by grade and uniformly, limiting buildup at the pinnacle plates (buildup can make the agar hard to appearance, and might turn out to be a vector for infection). A comparable effect

may be finished thru covering every stack with a spotless coffee cup or giant glass 1/2-loaded up with warmness water.

10. Permit plates to chill medium-time period.

eleven. Peroxide plates may be left for a few days in a fab sans draft spot to moreover pressure off any residual buildup. Lay them out in stacks of some, inexactly secured with a couple of sheets of clean waxed paper. Plates with out peroxide need to be located in sleeves when they have cooled.

12. Slide the plastic sleeve decrease again over the plates and tape it close firmly with smooth pressing tape. Store them agar element up (to moreover restrict buildup) in a cool and dry location until required.

Care of Petri Dishes and Cultures

When making transfers, lids want to be removed for as brief a time as may be anticipated beneath the situations, and held legitimately over the plate to preserve contaminants out.

Cultures ought to be stockpiled aspect up too. Be that as it could, it's far a outstanding plan to provide new transfers an afternoon or in order to develop out onto the modern day plate earlier than flipping around them, or the moved cloth probably may not preserve fast to the clean agar floor. Culture plates want to be wrapped round their edges with some layers of parafilm.

Spore Streaking

Even in case you use PF Tek to broaden P. Cubensis mushrooms or gather sparkling specimens from the wild, you can want to start your plants from spores to isolate a pressure of natural fruiting. There are strategies you may use to begin cultivation of mushrooms from spores to agar. A sterile inoculating loop is used in the traditional device to extract a small degree of the spores from a print, after which streaked over an agar plate. Remember which you can't use Petri plates containing peroxide because of this, as it would slaughter the spores. On the alternative thing, spores are sprouted in easy cardboard circles in an present day system advanced with the beneficial aid of Rush Wayne and illustrated in extent of his e-book Growing Mushrooms the Easy Way.

This approach gives a few unmistakable benefits over the conventional approach. The small size of the circles and the tight openings of the test tubes assist maintain contaminants out of cultures which may be unprotected thru peroxide. In addition, it's miles a absolutely rapid machine: the circles are proper away colonized and will then be able to be placed legitimately onto peroxidated agar.

Finally, due to the fact the circle demonstrations each due to the reality the substrate and due to the truth the tool used to reinforce spores from the spore print, it includes a talented trade, this is in particular beneficial when the spore print is black out and moderate on spores. Utilizing a punching tool, small circles are lessen from skinny, flat cardboard (the grey sheets placed inside the decrease lower back of stack of paper are awesome). These are moistened barely, positioned in a jar and sterilized along aspect check tubes containing 5-10 drops of a malt-yeast extract answer. At the component whilst cool, the circles are used to choose up a small quantity of spores, and later on dropped into the tube, in which they ingest the malt answer. In time, the spores expand and even as the modest circles are absolutely colonized, they're transferred to peroxide agar plates.

Agar Spore Germination

This method is indistinguishable from the simplest used at the same time as making spore-water syringes, other than that proper right here the spores are transferred to sans peroxide agar plates instead of water.

Materials

☐ Spore print

☐ Sans peroxide agar

☐ Petri dishes

☐ Inoculating loop

☐ Alcohol lamp

Parafilm

1. Heat the inoculation loop in the alcohol lamp to your glove discipline or waft hood till it sparks out outstanding-warm.

2. Using your specific hand to beautify the lid of the primary Petri dish, touch the give up of the loop to the point of interest of the agar to loosen up it (this moreover locations a skinny agar movie on the loop, as a way to permit the spores to stick to it).

3.   Cover the plate and in some time use the loop to choose up a small amount of spores from your print.

four.   Streak those throughout the Petri dish in a S-fashioned motion and in a while near the plate.

five.   Re-sterilize and cool the loop earlier than marking each plate.

6.   Wrap the rims of every plate with parafilm after inoculation, mark them with any applicable data, and hatch agar aspect up.

Cardboard Disk Spore Germination

Materials

☐   Spore print

☐   Cardboed circles

☐   J 2 pint jar and lid Screw-capped test tubes or vials (2 or 3 for every spore print)

☐   Malt yeast agar answer (1 tsp malt and a little pinch of yeast extract in 1 00 mL water)

☐   Pipette or eyedropper

☐   Tweezers

☐   Alcohol lamp

Parafilm

1.   Place cardboard circles in J/2-pint jar, along with 1 - 2m1 water, and seal. Place five-10 drops of malt solution into take a look at tubes and gently seal. Sterilize the jar and tubes for 15 minutes at forty five psi and permit to kick back in fact.

2.   Place your glove challenge or waft hood with all of the machine and materials.

3.   Heat the alcohol lamp tweezers up to excessive and permit to sit back.

4.   Open the jar and extract one circle the usage of tweezers. Spread jar.

five.　Lightly touch the edge of the circle to a part of the spore print. You should have the choice to look the black spores protective fast to the plate.

6.　Open a take a look at tube and drop the plate onto the lowest of the tube.

7.　Repeat 3-five times for every tube.

eight.　Create in any occasion tubes of plates for every spore print.

9.　Seal the tubes with parafilm and hatch.

10. At the issue even as the spores have sprouted and the circles are really colonized, circulate a pair to singular peroxide-containing agar plates.

Incubation

Vaccinated subculture plates and spore circles ought to be hatched in a warmth, sans draft region, inside the seventy five-eighty five° F range. In the occasion that the temperature in your private home is constantly inside this range, at that factor it is good sufficient to virtually keep them in an amazing discipline.

Tissue Transfers (Cloning)

Clean, glowing, mushrooms, either fruited from a multispore subculture (from a PF Tek jar, for example), or gathered from the wild, can likewise be used to begin an agar manner of life. Right now, coming approximately manner of lifestyles should be a solitary strain and must display indistinguishable attributes from its determine. Since it's far hereditarily indistinguishable from the stress from which it turn out to be secluded, it's miles regarded as a clone, and this technique is called cloning. Because of this, we generally look for the healthiest specimens in a population to clone, with the choice of putting aside a pressure in an effort to supply everyday and dynamic fruitings with every use. Good characters to look for in a discern incorporate early, huge, or thick quit end result, and any that have a healthy appearance in well-known. Isolating a solitary, fruiting strain is as primary as deciding on the most specimens out of your yields and culturing them on agar.

The mushrooms are torn or lessen open in a glove field or glide hood, and a small piece of smooth mycelium is eliminated from the inner of the stipe or the area of the cap without a doubt over the gills and positioned on a glowing agar plate. After a short brooding duration, the mycelial fragments grow out onto the plate and could then be capable of be subcultured. Often however the reality that, for unknown reasons, clones taken from a similar discern mushroom do display diverse mycelial traits.

Consequently, we make numerous (at the least four) cultures from all of us, and spare definitely the fine coming about cultures for added use. Looks can be beguiling and contours won't perform as expected via manner of way in their appearance, so we clone the equal enormous sort of various specimens as time and area permits, as a way to decorate our opportunities of achievement over the extended haul. Because they've got in no way been uncovered to the outer state of affairs, the cells on the internal of a mushroom ought to be clean (i.E., uncontaminated). To make certain sterility, be that as it is able to, you want to commonly attempt to clone mushrooms at the earliest possibility inside the wake of selecting them. If you can't use them immediately, you may keep them inside the ice chest in a smooth Tupperware area consistent with a sparkling paper towel for multiple days, but very little longer. Unlike on the equal time as streaking spores, peroxide inside the agar media will clearly beautify your possibilities of effective cloning, as it offers a in addition layer of safety from contaminants. Accordingly, we strongly endorse utilizing peroxidated agar at some thing element doing tissue cultures, except if you find out that the species or pressure being said does not tolerate it.

Tissue Transfers

Materials Mushroom(s)

☐ Petri dishes (with peroxide)

☐ Scalpel

☐ Alcohol

☐ Alcohol lamp

☐ Cotton balls or paper towel

1.   Before use, mushrooms for cloning want to be wiped smooth without a doubt of any free casing cloth. If viable 2 this way want to be completed a ways from the administrative center. Preferably dealing with an alcohol-soaked cotton ball in your glove situation or go along with the drift hood cleans the mushroom's outer surfaces.

2.   Sterilize the alcohol lamp with scalpel. Press the mushroom delicately among your

thumb and index finger, shielding it at the base of the stipe. You ought to have the choice to divide it alongside the centerline, and then strip the mushroom's halves divided the lengthy manner, if possible, truely thru the cap. If it is a small instance, or isn't parting successfully, you may use the scalpel alternatively to open it. Try to keep away from permitting the blade to legally contact the region from which you need to clone, as it is able to pose pollution on your life-style at the outer surfaces of the mushroom.

three.   After each use, sterilize the cutting thing another time.

four.   Cut a small piece of mycelium from an much less expensive place of the stipe or cap (usually on the thickest, most thickly packed place) along facet your Petri dishes equipped. It want to be as huge a piece as is probably anticipated underneath the instances, ideally from three-8 mm large and extended. Be especially cautious not to reduce right via to the mushroom's unsterile outer layers.

5.   Lance the mycelium fragment gently onto your scalpel end. Lift the Petri dish lid in your precise hand, area the fragment inside the middle of the agar and near the plate afterwards. (Sometimes the stringy concept of the mycelium will motive it to stick to the prevent of the pointy fringe of the scalpel; assuming that is the case, take a slice to reduce thru the fragment and push it down into the agar as you are doing as such.)

6.   Repeat with at least three plates for each mushroom.

7.   Seal the plates with parafilm, mark them nicely, and place them for your hatchery. Store them at once up till they begin to broaden out, and in some time turn round them now not extraordinarily. You need to start to see growth inner a couple of days to seven days. From the begin, the

fragment will turn out to be uniformly fluffy, as its cells start to isolate yet again; in the end the mycelium will fan out from in which it contacts the agar to colonize the complete plate.

Agar-to-Agar Transfers (Sub culturing)

A small piece of healthful-searching mycelium from the edge of a crop is reduce out with a sterile scalpel and positioned on the center of another plate to make agar-to-agar transfers. Growing cultures ought to be used or subcultured in advance than the mycelium receives too close to the brink of the plate, due to the truth the outer edges of the plate will harbor pollutants, which may be blanketed under the contemporary mycelial the front, most effective to develop on the identical time as they will be moved to each one-of-a-kind media.

Any a part of the propelling thing could be subcultured within the event the society is a mere pressure. If it is a multi-stress lifestyle (as an example, that rising from multispore inoculation), then you'll want to pick out mycelium with the best attributes at that detail. The presence of at the least forms of mycelia within a solitary community is referred to as sectoring. The visible look of a strong stress varies in addition from species to species, however thick rhizomorphic improvement for all Psilocybe species is a excellent sign of current health. Consider divisions with slight growth or wispy-looking mycelium which may be loads tons less probably to provide a pressure of fruiting.

Also placed the agar wedge face down on the clean plate, at the same time as creating a go with the flow. That serves   vital capacities. Above all, it brings the mycelium in direct touch with the agar, advancing the state-of-the-art plate's fast colonization. Furthermore, via sandwiching the mycelium among layers of agar containing peroxide, any contaminant spores or micro-organisms that keep away at the mycelial floor are destroyed.

Agar-to-Agar Transfers

Materials

☐   Agar manner of lifestyles (s)

☐   Sterile agar plates

☐   Scalpel Alcohol lamp

Parafilm

1.   In a glove box or drift hood, eliminate any parafilm from the outdoor of your wholesome manner of existence dish.

2.   Heat the threshold of the scalpel on your alcohol lamp till it gleams, at that aspect cool it in a clean Petri dish.

three.   Holding the lid of the primary lifestyle dish slightly, reduce squares or wedges of agar and mycelium from the proper segments of the plate, from 1/2 of to one centimeter tremendous. For the best of simplicity, you can reduce greater than each wedge in turn.

four.   To make the transfer, you have to do away with the lid of the number one way of lifestyles plate completely. With the blade in a unmarried hand, deliver the lid of an appropriate plate slightly to the alternative aspect, skewer one wedge of agar from the way of life plate at the tip of the blade and location it at the middle of the modern-day plate, mycelium element down.

five.   Repeat on all plates, seal and imprint truly, and region within the hatchery, the opportunity manner up no longer highly. (Wedges of agar stick properly to easy agar, permitting the plates to be altered proper away.)

Contamination

Contamination in cultivation of mushrooms is inescapable. One of the blessings of running with the two-dimensional agar plate ground is that pollution are without problems detected and remoted from balanced cultures. Plates which provide a few indication of contamination need to be eliminated from the growing vicinity and right away discarded.

Every so often, it might be critical to try to "salvage" a debased manner of life (in the event that you usually do more than one indistinguishable transfers and preserve easy art work propensities, such events should be pretty uncommon.) In this example, you want to constantly bypass the life-style away from its contaminants to every specific plate. In the event that you try and get rid of contaminants from an agar dish thru reducing the intruders from the plate, you'll likely really spread the contamination further. Because shape spores are so handily dissatisfied, it's miles specially hard to keep away from moving contaminants together together with your way of lifestyles to new plates and may take a few transfers before they will be simply disposed of.

Diagnosing the Sources of Contamination on Agar

You can frequently decide the deliver of contaminants on agar via looking the instance of the contamination at the plate.

1.   If contamination indicates up in advance than the plates are used, it thoroughly may be a signal of missing disinfection of the agar, terrible sterile method at some stage in pouring or potential of the plates, or an inadequate convergence of peroxide inside the medium.

2.   If signs of contamination arise on the outrageous edges of the plate, both in singular settlements or in an entire ring, it may display that non-sterile air had been drawn into the plates as they cooled. To save you this, permit the agar cool efficiently in advance than pouring it, and

spread the plates with their plastic sleeve immediately inside the wake of filling them.

3.   Contamination starting on the inoculation issue technique that each a debased discern life-style or bad cleaning of the blade or inoculation loop. Look at cultures to be transferred carefully earlier than using them and keep away from the use of any which may be suspect. Always warmth inoculating equipment until they spark sizzling.

4.   Bacterial contamination suggests up as disgusting, glowing, translucent roundabout provinces, frequently white, crimson, or yellow in shade. Microbes thrive in wet conditions and are effects spread onto plates with overabundance buildup on their lids. Always maintain up until agar has cooled because it ought to be before pouring, permit plates cool often of their plastic sleeve, and keep them agar element up.

Long-Term Strain Storage

When you have were given disengaged a healthy fruiting stress, you could need some manner to unfold this equal stress for a long term, with the intention that you do now not need to constantly repeat the detachment approach. Cloning from plate to plate again and again will in the end reason the strain to senesce, regardless of whether or no longer you alter your agar recipe continuously, as we endorse. Along those traces, you constantly need to apply cultures which have been uncovered to as slightly any transfers as may be predicted under the circumstances. To try this, you need to create an "ace" subculture of any pressure you keep in mind deserving of proliferation, as speedy you distinguish it. The ace life-style is then positioned into refrigerated, prolonged-time period stockpiling, and subcultured diverse. Cultures which can be stored at widespread fridge temperatures (38° F) input a circumstance of suspended animation and can be restored via using clearly sub culturing them to a clean plate. After a quick restoration duration, the lifestyle will keep normal boom. We advise setting away cultures on sterilized paper pellets in take a look at tubes. Strains saved on agar can prevent to exist all of the unexpected, probably inferable from the immoderate sugar content material cloth of the media. The healthy content material of paper is insignificant, however reputedly ok to preserve the manner of life healthy for lengthy durations.

The limited mouths of test tubes are ideal for ' proscribing buildup and infection, and their small length takes into attention smooth capability. However, in the occasion which you do now not method check tubes, you may use half of-pint mason jars or distinct similar small autoclavable packing containers. In the wake of shifting the tradition to the tube and allowing it to develop out, the tubes are placed in an auxiliary area, (for instance, a Ziploc bag) and saved within the refrigerator. Strains saved along the ones strains can stay realistic for a long term, but it's miles a extremely good plan to get better cultures intermittently (while constantly or) via manner of sub culturing every to a plate, at that component coming back to sparkling paper for added capability. The results of peroxide on cultures stored for lengthy durations aren't fantastic and ultimately we maintain it reduce unfastened our capacity media.

Paper Pellet Storage Medium

Materials

☐ Paper pellet tom cat clutter

☐ Faucet water Test tubes or one of a kind low priced bins

A channel

1.   Moisten paper pellets to location capacity.

2.   Burden internal pipe, absolute' 10' /2. Be vigilant to avoid any medium bits from the outside of the tubing. Seal for free of charge.

3.   Put the containers in your stress cooker and sterilize in layers for 1/2-hour at 15 psi. Jars, at the same time as check tubes need to be set up a rack or a wire to hold them upright.

4.   At the point whilst the cooker has come decrease again to atmospheric pressure but remains warmth to touch, open it, and punctiliously switch the boxes on your glove field and allow to take a seat again.

Inoculating Storage Tubes

Paper pellet tubes are vaccinated in addition to Petri dishes. Because the cultures lack peroxide, and they're presupposed to be stored so long as feasible, you have to take additional care to keep away from providing contaminants at the identical time as doing as such, following all the identical vintage precautions. In addition, you need to sterilize the neck of the inclination tube each time it is opened, with the resource of moving it internal the fireplace of your alcohol lamp.

1.   Fire the scalpel and the neck of the open tube.

2.   Cut a small piece of agar out of a wholesome lifestyle and positioned it inside the tube of the sawdust. Since the check tube necks are too confined to even do not forget permitting the blade to penetrate, it's miles less complicated to maintain the tube on a degree plane, area the wedge on the higher mass of the tube, seal it, after which thump it onto the sawdust delicately in some time.

three.　　Seal the jar, cover the cap or lid with a parafilm band and print it out properly.

four.　　Hatch till the paper is really colonized, at that element location the tubes into an optionally to be had region, for example, a cooler bag or Tupperware container and refrigerate.

Recovering Cultures from Storage

To get better a way of lifestyles from its stockpiling discipline, go back the tradition to room temperature for 48 hours, and switch (under the standard smooth situations) a small chunk of mycelium-secured paper from the ability field to a smooth, peroxidated agar Petri dish.

Chapter 16: Fruiting bins

Wbird you have got were given a totally colonized substratum, it must be put in a suitable subject for casing and fruiting. The field you choose relies upon on the amount of substrate to be fruited and may range from a small aluminum foil bread dish to a massive receptacle for plastic transport. You will give interest to 2-three inches of substratum intensity whilst fruiting smaller portions of grain, and as a bargain as 6 inches for big portions. Besides scale, on the identical time as selecting a fruiting difficulty, there are fantastic competencies to preserve in mind. It ought to be made from a fabric that is adequately unbending to preserve the substratum in vicinity as it colonizes, and it want to be truely opaque, allowing you to absorb slight on my own at the ground of the casing soil. Furthermore, the container's absolute depth want to as an alternative be close to doubling the substratum depth to permit clean alternate of gasoline even as starting up the sphere for misting.

For example, some growers use smaller, without a doubt enclosed containers, plastic canisters with Snap-On spreads to create a moist surroundings. While this does artwork, it calls for reducing or drilling holes inside the discipline elements to allow exchange of gasoline, and it ensures that the top must be transparent at any charge to allow slight to fall on the surface of the shell. Alternatively, we recommend the usage of shallower, opaque bins which might be then positioned inside the clammy, a fruiting chamber's sufficiently awesome setting.

The fruiting chamber can be as straightforward as an unmistakable plastic bag perforated to permit change of fuel, located nearly a sunlit window, or as complex as a multi-layered shelf tool that holds multiple containers, equipped with synchronized blinding lighting and a humidification.

The varieties of fruiting packing containers that we regularly use are plastic dishwasher tubes, 1 1.Five"x thirteen.5"x five "massive, which maintain 4-eight vicinity jars or one bag of grain, or 20"x Is" X 7 "deep plastic packing containers for big portions of substrates. The smaller dishpans are furnished in gadget and kitchen supply shops, and the conveyor receptacles can in fashionable be presented at the café deliver war.

The Humidity Tent

The cased bins have to be stored in a damp environment to save you fast lack of dampness from the casing and substrate. Unlike severa special cultivated mushrooms that require large stages of relative humidity (ninety%-a hundred%), we've got got positioned that Psilocybe cubensis does amazing and dandy with plenty lower levels (proper down to 70%).As prolonged as the sector is located in a nook that is sufficiently small, and the casing soil is stored very lots watered, sufficient water will wick into the immediately environment to preserve the mushrooms glad.. Smaller plate or tubs can in reality be placed into easy plastic luggage and tied shut.

Holes have to be punched or reduce inside the pinnacle and aspects of the bag to reflect onconsideration on gas trade, with 4 or five half of of of-inch holes normal with square foot. (A few on-line mushroom carriers sell pre-perforated luggage precisely for this motive.) The field need to be eliminated from the bag sooner or later of misting to assist displace amassed carbon dioxide. The baggage must be sufficiently huge to oblige the developing mushrooms, that permits you to increase as lots as 8 inches over the pinnacle of the casing soil.

Larger single containers may be located interior rearranged clear plastic storage tubes, with holes bored for gas exchange of their facets, or located on a tented shelf body. A type of lawn supply catalogs and online shops promote "growing racks". These are 3 or four-layered moderate-weight racks enclosed internal a zippered plastic tent for moisture manage. At the point while those make exceptional character mushroom developing fenced in areas whilst combined with a controlled lights tool. Can shelf can keep a few smaller boxes or one transportation tank, with lots of area to residence the growing mushrooms in among every shelf.

Humidity Levels

Small fruiting packing containers need to go into perforated plastic baggage, single big ones need to bypass into large baggage or smooth tubs, and more than one massive ones can be positioned on an encased broaden rack. For some component time period that the dimensions of the humidity chamber is firmly matched to the amount of substrate it consists of, the dampness tiers internal must be in reality easy to preserve up with a greater than as quickly as consistent with day hand misting.

At the point at the same time as the casing soil is all spherical watered, it want to wick sufficient water into the at once surroundings to preserve the growing mushrooms pleased. In the occasion that the air to your growing area takes place to be mainly dry, you can want to fall again on a beneficial humidification tool. Right now, least for the small-to-medium scale grower, the extraordinary scale is a fab mist (Impeller) style humidifier, which does no longer use warmth to create humidity and, in this manner, might not superfluously improve the temperatures of your trimming area. These are modest and with out troubles available at maximum huge pharmacies and retail chains.

We have visible extremely good growers expand entangled tubing structures for siphoning soggy air from a humidifier proper right right into a develop rack. This is probably important at the identical time as fruiting massive numbers of packing containers one after every other, however in great the humidifier itself can clearly be positioned on one of the racks along the plate. Buildup will growth on the dividers of the enclosure, so it is a top notch plan to location a large plate under the rack to defend dampness from falling legitimately onto the floor. Unfilled and smooth this plate often to keep away from shape improvement.

Lighting

Your lighting fixtures setup must likewise be scaled virtually for your fruiting region. Psilocybe mushrooms are not like plants of their lights requirements. They use mild simply to animate growth, not as a power supply, and they virtually require short day by day times of it to fruit successfully. A right well-known guiding principle is that if the gap is lit correctly to see properly, it should assist fruiting quality and dandy. A couple PF Jars or a solitary bath may want to require minimal in extra of a south-effective window or right encompassing electric powered powered lights. Larger increase racks could require an inherent lights setup.

We have positioned that 15-20-watt conservative colorful light bulbs paintings dependably well and use nearly no energy.

However, they should be installed outdoor the amplify chamber (probable mounted to a contiguous divider) to restrict heating and reduce the hazard of an electrical short out.

Depending on the dimensions and quantity of boxes in the enclosure, it might be critical to mount lamps at some regions if you need to avoid throwing shadows at the cultures. Electric lighting fixtures structures must likewise be positioned on timers, set to enlighten the gap for eight hours out of each day.

Chapter 17: Casing soil

Most cultivated species of mushrooms, like Psilocybe cubensis, can yield wealthy fruit best if the substratum is covered in a soil-like layer known as a casing layer. For instance, peat moss or vermiculite, on the thing of gypsum and calcium carbonate, are normally composed of non-nutritious substances with excessive water-retaining capacities. The casing layer serves some of important mushrooms producing capacities. The coating is supporting to shield the substratum from dropping its moisture to the environment due to its high-water content material cloth. It offers a moist microenvironment indoors which the touchy primordia can increase, and it serves as a water-saving to attract at the parched mushrooms as they broaden. Since the case layer takes up and discharges water like a wash, it moreover permits a grower to hold a mattress effortlessly at its perfect degree of moisture thus lowering the hazard of waterlogging the substratum and suffocating the fungus.

Furthermore, the amount of moisture on the particulate casing layer is regularly a whole lot much less complicated to "capture" than on uncovered colonized soil, thereby enhancing the humidification method. Many recipes for the casing soil encompass mineral salts, which include chalk and gypsum. To a few diploma, peat moss is acidic, and mushroom mycelium frequently oozes acidic metabolites as they broaden. Since a quite acidic surroundings can damage the fungus and useful resource the increase of microscopic organisms, the addition of chalk (calcium carbonate) to the casing soil permits to hold a slightly critical situation (a pH of 7.Five-eight.Five). Gypsum (calcium sulfate) is delivered to help preserve a unfastened, vaporous structure, and provide the growing fungus with mineral sustenance as calcium and sulfur. Assumed "water crystals" are arbitrary fixations that you can observe in your casing combination. Made of a artificial polymer chemically associated with exquisite paste, these crystals can assimilate 4 hundred times their weight in water, after which slowly discharge it back into their surroundings. They look like crisp gelatin while completely hydrated.

They are used to show water use in agriculture and gardening, and to protect plant life from drying out really amongst watering. Similarly, the addition to a casing layer of most effective a small amount of water crystals might serve to maintain it hydrated and reduce the need for regular misting. A unmarried flush of mushrooms will ransack a big quantity of water from the casing and substratum, and these crystals can give your cultures a further degree of protection from drying out. Despite being a artificial substance, water crystals were examined and tested to be non-unstable and kindhearted to the environment. We really convert to carbon dioxide and water after some time. We have even been experimentally tested for safety while implemented in developing mushrooms. Catch mushrooms (Agaricus bisporus) grown of their presence have not been proven to deprave or introduce the gel's chemical factors.

The crystals are to be had assortments: ones made from sodium or others crafted from potassium. Since incredible ranges of sodium are dangerous to severa fungi, ensure to get the sort crafted from potassium. Because the crystals debase at the same time as heated, they want to be added in the wake of disinfecting or sanitizing the casing soil. While a few growers advocate sanitizing casing soils in advance than use to restrict contaminations, we have discovered this development useless as long as the components are stored perfect and dry within the first place. Nonetheless, within the occasion which you need to be more careful or you discover that you do experience trouble with contamination in your casing, a brisk sanitization may also furthermore assist. A number one approach for sanitizing small portions uses a microwave oven. Simply area the sodden, Prepared container soil in a heat-evidence field or bag (large oven bags, the kind used to prepare dinner turkeys, or huge plastic cooler baggage are perfect) and microwave it on excessive for approximately 15 mins. Make fantastic the bag or bottle is left unsealed to keep away from blasting. Enable the bag to sit for 10 mins, then microwave for every other 15 mins afterwards. If you do no longer have a microwave, you can additionally sterilize it at 15 psi for forty five mins in a stress cooker or prepare it for 2 hours in a 3500 oven. Before the use of allow to relax without a doubt. You may additionally want to feature more water to repair the casing soil to region potential, because it will absolutely force some moisture off after heating. We've furnished 3 smooth casing recipes, simply to offer you a experience of the sorts used and to leverage the belongings which you might probable have with out trouble to be had.

www.ingramcontent.com/pod-product-compliance
Lightning Source LLC
Chambersburg PA
CBHW062141020426
42335CB00013B/1298